Emergency Maternity Care

T0195475

For Elsevier
Content Strategist: Alison Taylor
Content Development Specialist: Veronika Watkins
Project Manager: Julie Taylor
Designer: Paula Catalano
Illustration Manager: Amy Faith Heyden

VOLUME **6**

MIDWIFERY ESSENTIALS

Emergency Maternity Care

Helen Baston, BA(Hons), MMedSci, PhD, PGDipEd, ADM, RN, RM
Consultant Midwife Public Health;
Sheffield Teaching Hospitals,
NHS Foundation Trust, UK;
Honorary Researcher/Lecturer, University of Sheffield;
Honorary Lecturer, Sheffield Hallam University, UK

Jenny Hall, EdD, MSc, RN, RM, ADM, PGDip(HE), SFHEA, FRCM
Senior Lecturer, Centre for Excellence in Learning,
Bournemouth University, UK

Contributions from Alison Brodrick, MSc, RN, RM, DipHE
Consultant Midwife, Sheffield Teaching Hospitals NHS
Foundation Trust, UK
Honorary Lecturer University of Sheffield

ELSEVIER

Edinburgh London New York Oxford Philadelphia St Louis Sydney Toronto 2018

ELSEVIER

ISBN 978-0-7020-7102-7
e_ISBN 978-0-7020-7152-2

Notices
Practitioners and researchers must always rely on their own experience and knowledge in evaluating and using any information, methods, compounds or experiments described herein. Because of rapid advances in the medical sciences, in particular, independent verification of diagnoses and drug dosages should be made. To the fullest extent of the law, no responsibility is assumed by Elsevier, authors, editors or contributors for any injury and/or damage to persons or property as a matter of products liability, negligence or otherwise, or from any use or operation of any methods, products, instructions, or ideas contained in the material herein.

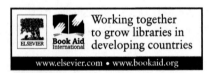

Working together
to grow libraries in
developing countries

www.elsevier.com • www.bookaid.org

your source for books,
journals and multimedia
in the health sciences

www.elsevierhealth.com

The
publisher's
policy is to use
**paper manufactured
from sustainable forests**

Printed in Great Britain

Last digit is the print number: 10 9 8 7 6 5 4 3 2

Contents

Preface

To contribute to the provision of sensitive, safe and effective maternity care for women and their families is a privilege. Childbirth is a life-changing event for women. Those around them and those who have an input into any aspect of pregnancy, labour, birth or the postnatal period can positively influence how this event is experienced and perceived. To achieve this, maternity carers continually need to reflect on the services they provide and strive to keep up-to-date with developments in clinical practice. They should endeavour to ensure that women are central to the decisions made and that real choices are offered and supported by skilled practitioners.

This book is the sixth volume in a series of texts based on the popular 'Midwifery Basics' series published in *The Practising Midwife* journal. The books have remained true to the original style of the articles and have been updated and expanded to create a user-friendly source of information. They are also intended to stimulate debate and require readers both to reflect on their current practice, local policies and procedures and to challenge care that is not woman-centred. The use of scenarios enables practitioners to understand the context of maternity care and explore their role in its safe and effective provision.

There are many dimensions to the provision of woman-centred care that practitioners need to consider and understand. To aid this process, a jigsaw model has been introduced, with the aim of encouraging readers to explore maternity care from a wide range of perspectives. For example, how does a midwife obtain consent from a woman for a procedure, maintain a safe environment during the delivery of care and make the most of the opportunity to promote health? What are the professional and legal issues in relation to the procedure, and is this practice based on the best available evidence? Which members of the multi-professional team contribute to this aspect of care, and how is it influenced by the way care is organized? Each aspect of the jigsaw should be considered during the assessment, planning, implementation and evaluation of woman-centred maternity care.

Midwifery Essentials: Emergency Maternity Care is about the provision of safe and effective care when the birth process deviates from normal. It reflects the focus of the National Maternity Review, *Better Births* (2016) endorsing personalized care and real choice for women. It comprises 11 chapters, each written to stand alone or be read in succession. The introductory chapter sets the scene, exploring the role of the midwife in the context of professional and national guidance. The jigsaw model for midwifery care is introduced and explained, providing a framework to explore each aspect of emergency care, described in subsequent chapters. Chapter 2 explores the care of a woman who experiences antepartum haemorrhage. Bleeding in pregnancy is a frightening event for women, filling them with fear that they may lose their baby. The prompt and sensitive response by the midwife will make a difference to her experience and the potential outcome of this event. Chapter 3 focuses on the care of the baby in the period immediately after birth and how the midwife can take steps to initiate effective resuscitation if required. Chapter 4 describes the care of a woman whose baby presents by the breech and her role within the multi-professional team to provide a skilled and competent response. Chapter 5 focuses on the recognition and immediate care of a woman who experiences shoulder dystocia. Chapter 6 examines the causes and responses to postpartum haemorrhage, including the management of retained placenta. In Chapter 7 the role of the midwife in the care of a woman with eclampsia, both in the antenatal and postpartum periods, is discussed. In Chapter 8, the recognition and management of psychiatric emergencies is described, including the contributions of the wider multi-disciplinary team. In Chapter 9, a range of uterine emergencies is presented including uterine prolapse, uterine inversion and scar dehiscence. Chapter 10 focuses on cord complications and the book concludes with Chapter 11, which discusses the recognition, and management of sepsis. This book thoroughly prepares the reader to provide safe, evidence-based, woman-centred emergency care for mothers and their babies.

National Maternity Review (2016). *Better Births. Improving outcomes of maternity services in England.* Available at: https://www.england.nhs.uk/wp-content/uploads/2016/02/national-maternity-review-report.pdf

Sheffield and Bournemouth 2018

Helen Baston
Jennifer Hall

Acknowledgements

In the process of writing there are always people behind the scenes who support or add to the development of the book. We would specifically like to thank Mary Seager, formerly Senior Commissioning Editor at Elsevier, for her initial vision, support and prompting to turn the journal articles from *The Practising Midwife* into a readable volume. This project has now further developed as a result of the insight and patience of Veronika Watkins and Alison Taylor. In addition, neither of us could have completed this edition without the love, support and endless patience of our amazing families. To you we owe our greatest gratitude.

This edition also benefits from the valuable contributions of Alison Brodrick, Consultant Midwife, Sheffield Teaching Hospitals, NHS Foundation Trust.

CHAPTER 1

Introduction

Part 1: Introduction to the jigsaw model

This book is the sixth in the *Midwifery Essentials* series aimed at student midwives and those who support them in clinical practice. It focuses on emergency care for women and babies, beginning in this chapter with the principles of caring for a woman who has collapsed, followed by Chapter 2 describing care after antepartum haemorrhage. It then considers care of the neonate who requires resuscitation immediately after the birth, followed by how to care for the mother and fetus when the presentation is breech. The need for quick and effective action when shoulder dystocia occurs is then described; subsequently the management of postpartum haemorrhage and retained products of conception is considered. How to care for a woman who has an eclamptic fit is the focus of Chapter 7, followed by recognition in Chapter 8 of the distressing presentation of psychiatric emergencies, which require urgent care. Then obstetric emergencies involving the uterus are described in Chapter 9, followed by how to act when the umbilical cord presents or prolapses. The book concludes with how to recognize and manage a woman who is suffering from sepsis. Scenarios are used throughout the book to facilitate learning and assist the reader to apply this knowledge to her own practice areas. The focus for contemporary maternity care is choice, access and continuity of care within a safe and effective service (Department of Health 2004, 2007) where women receive information to choose a model of care that meets their personal needs (National Maternity Review 2016). This book explores ways in which this aspiration can become a reality for women and their families, even when care does not go according to plan.

The aim of this introductory chapter is:

Part 1: To introduce the 'jigsaw model' for exploring effective midwifery practice.

Part 2: To introduce the principles of caring for a collapsed woman.

The jigsaw model is used throughout the book with a view to helping midwives apply their knowledge in the provision of emergency care to women and their babies.

Midwifery care model

One of the purposes of this series of books is to consider the care of women and their babies from a holistic viewpoint. This means considering the care within a physical, emotional, psychological, spiritual, social and cultural context. To do this we have developed a jigsaw model of care (Fig. 1.1) that will encourage the reader to consider individual aspects of midwifery care, while recognizing that these aspects go to make up part of the whole person being cared for.

This model will be used to reflect on the clinical scenarios described in the chapters. It shows the dimensions of effective maternity care, and each should be considered during the assessment, planning, implementation and evaluation of an aspect of care.

The pieces of the jigsaw clearly interlink with each other, and each is needed for the provision of safe, holistic emergency care. When one is missing the picture will be incomplete and care will not reach its potential. Each aspect of the model is described in the text that follows in more detail. It is recommended that when an aspect of midwifery care is being evaluated each piece of the jigsaw is addressed. Consider the questions pertaining to each piece of the jigsaw and work through those that are relevant to the clinical situation you face.

Woman-centred care

The provision of woman-centred care was one of the central messages of the policy document *Changing Childbirth* (Department of Health 1993), which turned the focus of maternity care from meeting the needs of the

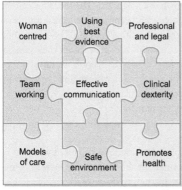

Fig. 1.1 Jigsaw model: dimensions of effective midwifery care.

professionals to listening and responding to the aspirations of women. This is further enforced in *Maternity Matters* (Department of Health 2007), *Better Births* (National Maternity Review 2016) and the National Institute for Health and Care Excellence (NICE) range of maternity-related guidance. The provision of woman-centred care is also an expectation of midwifery practice as prescribed by and preregistration education standards (NMC 2009). When considering particular aspects of care the questions that need to be addressed to ensure that the woman's care is woman-centred include:

- Was the woman involved in the development of her care plan and its subsequent implementation?
- How can I keep her informed of her progress during an emergency?
- How can I ensure that she remains involved in further decisions about her care?
- What are the implications of providing emergency care that is outside of her birth plan?
- Are there any personal factors that I need to consider that might influence the management of her care?
- How does the management of this emergency scenario fit in with the woman's hopes, expectations and beliefs?
- How do I involve her next of kin in decisions about her care management?

Using best evidence

A growing body of research evidence is available to inform the emergency care we provide. We have a duty to apply this knowledge, as the NMC Code states: 'always practice in line with the best available evidence' (NMC 2015: 7). The use of evidence in practice is complex and multifaceted, and its application is influenced by many factors, including its authority and consensus among colleagues (Kennedy et al 2012). Questions that need to be addressed when exploring the evidence base of care include:

- What is already known about this aspect of care?
- What is the justification for the choices made about care?
- What is the research evidence available on this procedure?
- Do local guidelines reflect best evidence?
- Was a midwife involved in development of local/national guidelines?
- Is there consensus among colleagues regarding best practice?
- Who represents users of maternity services on groups where guidelines are developed?
- What midwifery research projects has your Trust been involved in, in relation to emergency obstetric care?
- Where do you go first to identify sources of best evidence?

Professional and legal

Women need to feel confident that the midwives who care for them are working within a framework that supports safe practice. Midwives who practise in the UK must adhere to the guidance of the NMC. The Code (NMC 2015: 2) states:

> UK nurses and midwives must act in line with the Code, whether they are providing direct care to individuals, groups or communities or bringing their professional knowledge to bear on nursing and midwifery practice in other roles, such as leadership, education or research [...] This commitment to professional standards is fundamental to being part of a profession.

Midwives are therefore required to comply with English law and the rules and regulations of their employers.

Questions that need to be addressed to ensure that the woman's care fulfils statutory obligations include:

- Is this procedure expected to be an integral part of education before qualification?
- Which NMC proficiencies relate to this care?
- How does the NMC Code relate to this care?
- Is there any other NMC guidance applicable to this aspect of emergency care?
- Are there any national or international guidelines for this procedure?
- Are there any legal issues underpinning this aspect of care?

Team working

Although midwives are the experts in low-risk maternity care, they need to be robust in their response to an emergency situation and are reliant on a number of other workers to provide a comprehensive, safe service. Midwives work as part of a team of professional and support staff who each bring particular skills and perspectives to the care of women and their families. The NMC Code requires registrants to 'support students' and colleagues' learning to help them develop their professional competence and confidence' (2015: 9). It also states:

- respect the skills, expertise and contributions of your colleagues, referring matters to them when appropriate;
- maintain effective communication with colleagues;
- keep colleagues informed when you are sharing the care of individuals with other healthcare professionals and staff;
- work with colleagues to evaluate the quality of your work and that of the team;

- work with colleagues to preserve the safety of those receiving care;
- share information to identify and reduce risk; and
- be supportive of colleagues who are encountering health or performance problems. However, this support must never compromise or be at the expense of patient or public safety (NMC 2015: 8).

Questions that need to be addressed to ensure that appropriate use is made of the multiprofessional team in the woman's care include:

- Does this aspect of emergency care fall within my current role?
- Have I acknowledged the limitations of my professional knowledge?
- Who else will need to be involved in the provision of this care?
- Where is the most appropriate place to document this aspect of care?
- Who will I involve when observations of the woman are outside normal parameters?
- How can I facilitate effective team working with this woman?
- Will another person be required to assist with this aspect of emergency care?
- When will they be available and how can I access them?

Effective communication

Providing woman-centred care to women during an emergency situation requires midwives to engage and communicate effectively with them. It is essential that the midwife is aware of the cues she is giving to the woman during the care she provides. Time is often pressured in midwifery, both in the community and hospital setting, but it is important to convey to the woman that she is the focus of your attention. Taking time to explain what you are going to do and why is crucial if she is going to trust that you will always act in her best interest.

Questions that need to be addressed throughout postnatal care include:

- What opportunities are there for the woman to convey her hopes and fears?
- How can the midwife facilitate meaningful discussion about her choices for care?
- What information needs to be given to enable the woman to choose whether this is the right decision for her?
- How can the partner be effectively involved in supporting the woman during an emergency?
- Has she given consent for me to give this aspect of care?
- Does the woman understand what the care entails?
- In what ways could the information about this aspect of care be given?
- What should be said during the care?
- What should be observed in the woman's behaviour during the care?

+ What should be communicated to the woman after the care?
+ How and where should recording of the care and its effectiveness be made?

Clinical dexterity

Midwives providing emergency care need to exercise a range of skills to provide choices for women. They need to be able to employ competent technical knowledge when supporting a woman who is having a postpartum haemorrhage as well as using effective supportive and communication skills. Midwives need to apply their experience and wisdom to facilitate successful breech birth and have the confidence to encourage women to try alternative strategies when appropriate. The midwife continues to learn new skills throughout her working life and is accountable for maintaining and developing her practice as new ways of working are introduced, 'Keep your knowledge and skills up to date, taking part in appropriate and regular learning and professional development activities that aim to maintain and develop your competence and improve your performance' (NMC 2015: 17).

Questions that need to be addressed to ensure that the woman's care is provided with clinical dexterity include:
+ How has the emergency response changed since I first qualified as a midwife?
+ Can I provide this care in other ways?
+ How has my previous experience influenced how I approach this aspect of care today?
+ How can I be sure I am carrying this out correctly?
+ Are there opportunities for practising this skill elsewhere?
+ Whom can I observe to explore alternative ways of doing this?

Models of care

Midwives work in many settings and in a range of maternity care systems. For example, midwives work in primary care, providing care in women's homes, at drop-in clinics within general practitioner (GP) surgeries or in local children's centres. Midwives also work in a midwifery-led unit (MLU) providing holistic client-centred care, and within a large tertiary centre providing care for women with complex health needs. The models of care can be influential in determining the care that a woman may receive, from whom and when. Midwives need to consider the most appropriate ways that care can be delivered so that they can influence future development in the best interests of women and their families. Models of care are evolving in the light of the *Better Births* report (National Maternity Review 2016: 8), which states that women 'should be able to choose the provider of their antenatal, intrapartum and postnatal care'. A woman therefore needs to know what the response to an emergency might be in the place where she chooses to have her care. For example, what is the transfer time from the MLU to the obstetric unit, if she needed urgent care? What are the facilities available if the baby needed resuscitation at a home birth?

Questions that need to be addressed to ensure that the impact of the way that care is provided is acknowledged include:

+ How long has care been provided in this way?
+ How is the maternity service organized?
+ Which professional groups are involved in the provision of this service?
+ How is this procedure/care influenced by the model of care provided?
+ How does this model of care impact on the carers?
+ How does this model of care impact on the woman and her family?
+ Is this the best way to provide care from a professional point of view?
+ How is the woman facilitated to make choices about the care she has?

Safe environment

Midwives providing care need to ensure that the environment in which they work supports safe and effective working practices and protects the woman and her family from harm. The NMC Code states that 'You must maintain the knowledge and skills for safe and effective practice' (NMC 2015: 7). The midwife must ensure that the care she gives does not compromise the safety of women and their families. She must therefore create and maintain a safe working environment at all times, whether in a woman's home, children's centre or in a hospital service.

Questions that need to be addressed to ensure that the woman's care is provided in a safe environment include:

+ Does the woman understand the implications of giving her consent to this procedure?
+ Are there facilities to ensure that her privacy and dignity are maintained?
+ How will high standards of infection control be managed during this emergency?
+ Is there an appropriate place to dispose of waste?
+ Is the equipment appropriately maintained and free from contamination?
+ Is the space adequate to allow ease of movement around the woman in an emergency situation?
+ What are the risks involved in this procedure/care and how have they been addressed?

+   Are there any risks to the person undertaking this procedure/care?
+   Is this environment safe for others who might come into the room?

Promotes health

Providing emergency care for women and their babies saves lives and prevents potential morbidity through complications. It therefore presents a unique opportunity to influence their health and well-being. Midwives must capitalize on their contacts with women to help them achieve a positive adaptation to parenthood and ensure that they understand why a particular course of action was taken, to enable them to make appropriate choices in the future.

Questions that need to be addressed to ensure that the woman's care promotes health include:

+   Is this procedure/care going to help her or harm her or her baby in any way?
+   What are the opportunities after this emergency to educate her/her family on healthy behaviours?
+   What resources can women and families access to help them make healthy lifestyle choices?
+   Has enough time been allocated to this aspect of care to make the most of the opportunities to promote healthy living?
+   Who else should I involve to ensure that the woman and her family get the best possible advice after this situation?

The chapters use the jigsaw model (Fig. 1.1) to explore scenarios from practice, focusing on the role of the midwife in the various aspects of emergency care. Thus the reader is provided with a structure with which to reflect on her care and that of the multi-professional team in which she works. Each chapter includes a range of activities designed to enable the midwife to contextualize the information within her own practice, applying her continually developing knowledge to her own circumstances.

Part 2: Maternal collapse

Introduction

Most women embark on pregnancy anticipating a healthy journey to motherhood. Although this is usually the case, this path can be unpredictable and some women will become unwell and experience life-threatening complications. It is therefore essential that the healthcare professionals who care for pregnant and parturient women are skilled in the recognition and management of such conditions.

Definition and incidence

Maternal collapse has been defined as:

> 'an acute event involving the cardiorespiratory systems and/or brain, resulting in a reduced or absent conscious level (and potentially death), at any stage of pregnancy and up to six weeks after delivery'
>
> (Royal College of Obstetricians and Gynaecologists (RCOG) 2011: 2)

The maternal death rate in the UK is 8.8 per 100,000 (Knight et al 2017) although it is estimated that up to 100 times as many women experience significant complications leading to potential lifelong sequelae; the incidence of maternal collapse is estimated to be between 0.14 and 6 per 1000 births (Long & Penna 2018).

Another term that is also used in relation to maternal collapse is 'shock'. This occurs when a sudden drop in blood pressure results in underperfusion of the organs leading to hypoxia (lack of oxygen to the tissues).

Causes

There are many causes of maternal collapse (see Table 1.1), and it is therefore appropriate that the maternity care team have systems in place to predict and anticipate impending deterioration in the women in their care.

Prevention

It is recommended that a Modified Early Obstetric Warning Scoring system (MEOWS) is used to detect impending deterioration in the pregnant or postpartum woman (Singh et al 2012) (see Midwifery Essentials, Vol. 1:

Table 1.1: **Causes of maternal collapse**

Cause of collapse	Example of origin
Cardiovascular	Cardiac disease, congenital anomaly, syncope
Embolism	Thrombosis, amniotic fluid embolism
Sepsis	Infection: general and obstetric origins
Cerebrovascular	Stroke, epilepsy
Haemorrhage	Ruptured/ectopic uterus, trauma, brain, coagulopathy
Drug induced	Overdose, toxicity, withdrawal, anaphylaxis
Anaesthetic complications	Failed intubation, high central neuraxial block
Metabolic disorders	Hypoglycaemia, diabetic ketoacidosis
Seizure	Eclampsia, epilepsy

Basics). The MEOWS score alerts practitioners when to escalate their concerns about a woman for medical review and is based on undertaking and documenting maternal observations, including:

- Heart rate
- Respiration rate
- Oxygen saturation
- Blood pressure
- Temperature
- Mental state

Normal observations score zero, however, when maternal observations are outside normal parameters and depending on their degree of derangement, an objective warning score alerts the practitioner to a predefined course of action. It is important, however, that the clinical presentation is also taken into account and that a practitioner should not be reassured by a normal MEOWS if he or she is concerned about a woman's condition (Knight et al 2017).

Activity

Access the MEOWS where you work. In what circumstances are you required to complete a MEOWS for women in your care? What action would you need to take if a woman had a temperature of 37.8°C, a diastolic blood pressure reading of 60 mm Hg and a respiration rate of 17 breaths per minute?

Care of a collapsed woman
Background

Women with a significant medical or obstetric history should be cared for by a multi-professional team that can develop and implement a bespoke care plan; this team should include an experienced obstetric anaesthetist.

(Knight et al 2017: 71)

Because the nature of need for the team to work effectively together, it is recommended that they train together and that regular opportunities for practice, using simulation where possible, are made available (Smith et al 2012).

The role of the midwife

Although the midwife's remit is normality, she must also be able to act in an emergency until medical assistance arrives. She also needs to continue to support the care of the woman and ensure her relatives are being supported throughout the process of resuscitation.

The student midwife, learning about how to care for a woman who has collapsed, is familiarizing herself with the sequence of events and how to gain help. She may be called on to raise the alarm or to bring equipment and should familiarize herself with these life-saving activities in the first few days of her placement. She may be asked to escort other women on a ward to the next bay, so that they are not witnessing a distressing scene. Ultimately, her mentor is responsible for the care of the woman until medical aid arrives, but the student can learn a great deal from watching and listening to events as they unfold. A study of student midwives' experience of being involved in traumatic birth situations (Davis & Coldridge 2015) showed the student may be particularly vulnerable because of her close affiliation with the woman. Opportunity for reflection may help them understand the dynamics of their role and ultimately help them develop skills for self-care and build resilience (Coldridge & Davis 2017).

Assessing the situation

When a woman collapses unexpectedly, practitioners need to piece together information from the woman's history including:

- Previous and current medical history
- Previous and current obstetric history
- Previous and current social history
- Current clinical presentation
- Current observations and MEOWS

Previous and current medical history

For example, she may have a history of childhood asthma requiring hospitalization. Was there any note in her records that she had recently required treatment? Was she currently a smoker? What was her most recent carbon monoxide reading? Had she recently had a chest infection? Was there a possibility her respiratory arrest is asthma related?

OR

She may have a current history of allergy to penicillin, and this would require alerts on her case-notes, electronic patient records, drug cards and wrist labels. Had she been given any antibiotics earlier despite this knowledge? Was her collapse anaphylaxis?

Previous and current obstetric history

For example, she may have had a previous caesarean section and therefore have a scar on her uterus. Was there any evidence of fetal compromise or abdominal pain before she collapsed? Has she had a uterine rupture? Was this collapse due to haemorrhage?

OR

She may have a previous history of pre-eclampsia and induction of labour. Her latest diastolic blood pressure reading was 20 mm Hg above her booking reading, and a specimen of urine had been sent to the laboratory, as she was noted to have a proteinurea. Had any blood tests been requested? Is this an eclamptic seizure?

Previous and current social history

For example, she may have a history of previous drug misuse, self-harm and suicide attempts. What was her current mental health status? Had there been any significant events in this pregnancy? Had she disclosed that she was subject to domestic abuse? Had there been any recent toxicology screening? Was there a possibility she may have taken an overdose?

Current clinical situation

For example, had she recently given birth or complained of spontaneous rupture of membranes? Had she expressed a feeling of impending doom? Was she exhibiting restlessness, cyanosis or respiratory distress before she collapsed? Was there a possibility that she may have had an amniotic fluid embolism?

Current observations

For example, was there any evidence of infection or potential source of infection? Had she had her flu vaccination? Was she tachypnoeic on admission? Had her oxygen saturation been recorded? Was she hypotensive? Was there a possibility she could be in septic shock?

Activity

What are the symptoms of anaphylaxis? In what circumstances should the midwife be prepared for the possibility of an anaphylactic response? Where will you find an anaphylaxis drug box where you work (including community settings)?

Immediate response to maternal collapse

In the hospital setting it is likely that many of the tasks outlined in the text that follows and in Fig. 1.2 will take place simultaneously, depending on the size of the team and how quickly the resuscitation team arrives. For example, one person may be ringing for the resuscitation team, another

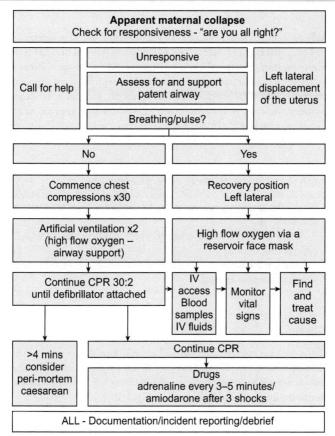

Apparent maternal collapse
Check for responsiveness - "are you all right?"

Call for help	Unresponsive
	Assess for and support patent airway
	Breathing/pulse?

Left lateral displacement of the uterus

No	Yes
Commence chest compressions x30	Recovery position Left lateral
Artificial ventilation x2 (high flow oxygen – airway support)	High flow oxygen via a reservoir face mask
Continue CPR 30:2 until defibrillator attached	IV access Blood samples IV fluids	Monitor vital signs	Find and treat cause

| >4 mins consider peri-mortem caesarean | Continue CPR |
| | Drugs adrenaline every 3–5 minutes/ amiodarone after 3 shocks |

ALL - Documentation/incident reporting/debrief

Fig. 1.2 Summary of actions after maternal collapse.

bringing the emergency trolley, another connecting the bag and mask to the oxygen supply, another cannulating her while another has started cardiac compressions. In the community setting, the midwife will commence basic life support procedures, until paramedic support arrives.

Safety

Ensure that it is safe to approach the woman, that there are no slip hazards/traffic as you walk towards her. If there are others nearby, ask someone to get help and/or call the emergency buzzer, if in a hospital setting.

Responsiveness

When a woman is found collapsed, her responsiveness should be determined by gently shaking her shoulders and asking loudly, 'Are you all right?' If she responds, then providing she is in a safe place and there is no evidence of injury, she should be put in the recovery position with her uterus displaced to the left. Medical attention should be sought and her observations recorded whilst a possible cause is being determined, for example, a faint (syncope) after giving a blood sample. Her condition should be regularly reassessed.

Activity

What is the emergency number to ring for the cardiac arrest team where you work?

Where is the resuscitation equipment kept on labour ward/antenatal clinic/postnatal ward?

How are the contents of the trolley checked and maintained, and who is responsible for this?

Airway

If she does not respond, turn her on her back, displace her uterus to her left and remove any pillows. Open her airway by simultaneously placing non-dominant hand on her forehead and tilting her chin upwards with dominant fore- and middle fingers (see Fig. 1.3).

Breathing

Check for signs of life – is she breathing? Look, listen and feel for signs of normal breathing, not gasping, for no more than 10 seconds. While doing so, check the carotid pulse. If she is not breathing or irregularly gasps, prepare to undertake cardiopulmonary resuscitation (CPR). Instruct any help that has arrived that the resuscitation team should be called immediately and that the resuscitation trolley with defibrillator should be brought.

If in the community, an emergency ambulance should be requested (999 in the UK), and if alone, select speaker mode on the phone.

Circulation

Chest compressions

Leaning directly over the woman, place the heel of the dominant hand in the centre of the chest (the middle of the lower half of the sternum). Place

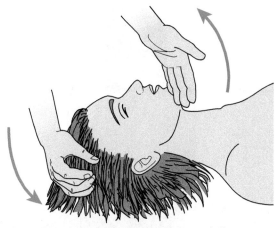

Fig. 1.3 Open airway. (With permission from Marshall J, Raynor M, eds., Myles Textbook for Midwives, 16th ed., p. 488, Fig. 22.12. Edinburgh: Churchill Livingstone/ Elsevier.)

the non-dominant hand on top of first hand and clasp fingers (see Fig. 1.4). The direction of downward pressure should be perpendicular to the chest wall, or a depth of 5 to 6 centimetres and at a rate of 100 to 120 per minute (Resuscitation Council UK 2015). Some people find it useful to have a tune in their head that enables them to perform at the correct rate, such as 'Nellie the elephant' or 'staying alive'. Deliver 30 uninterrupted chest compressions.

Activity

Find out about the different types of airway available where you work. How are they inserted and in what circumstances are they advocated?

Rescue breaths

After 30 chest compressions, two rescue breaths should be given. A two-person technique is most effective at a continued ratio of 30 chest compressions to 2 breaths, and they should swap roles every 2 minutes. Ventilation should preferably be given via a bag and mask with a reservoir bag and an oxygen supply. If help and equipment is still on its way, it may be necessary to perform mouth-to-mouth ventilation. This is achieved by pinching the nose with the non-dominant hand, lifting the chin with the dominant hand and placing the mouth over the mother's mouth and blowing for 1

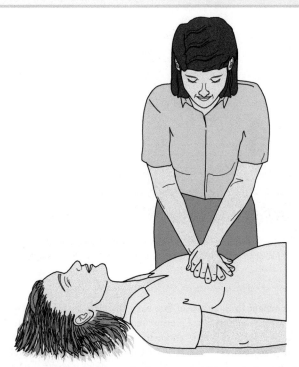

Fig. 1.4 Chest compression. (With permission from Marshall J, Raynor M, eds., Myles Textbook for Midwives, 16th ed., p. 488, Fig. 22.13. Edinburgh: Churchill Livingstone/Elsevier.)

second. An airway may be useful to maintain a patent airway, and the efficiency of the ventilation should be checked by observing for the chest rising. Then repeat as before and quickly return to cardiac compressions. It is important to use an oxygen-enriched air supply as soon as practical, as expired breath contains only up to 17% oxygen (RCOG 2011).

When the resuscitation team arrives, and if the woman is unconscious, their aim will be to intubate her as soon as possible. The additional weight of the baby and breast enlargement make ventilation less effective, especially in the third trimester (Long & Penna 2018). As she is at risk of aspiration of gastric contents, cricoid pressure should be used during intubation. When the woman has an endotracheal tube securely in place, her lungs should be ventilated at a rate of 10 breaths per minute, while chest compressions continue uninterrupted (Resuscitation Council UK 2015).

Use of a defibrillator

Many areas have automated external defibrillators (AEDs) which are simple to use. They can be attached before further help arrives and provide useful information about the patient's heart rhythm and whether or not it is shockable. Clear visual instructions show where to position the pads, and automated voice prompts guide even the untrained lay person to provide lifesaving treatment. CPR should be continued until just before the shock is delivered, and everyone should be clear from touching the patient to avoid inadvertent administration of a shock to a bystander. If a normal heart rhythm does not resume, CPR should be continued while the next administration is prepared for.

Fluids

While immediate CPR is in progress, another professional can be gaining venous access; two wide-bore cannulae should be inserted, one in each antecubital fossa. If blood tests are indicated, depending on the suspected primary cause of collapse, these should be quickly taken and then intravenous infusion (IVI) commenced. It is usual practice to infuse a crystalloid first, such as normal 0.9% saline or Hartman's solution, before recourse to a colloid. The aim is to maintain blood pressure and thus organ perfusion, but this must be carefully balanced and monitored, especially if pre-eclampsia is suspected.

Blood samples

Venous blood samples should be taken to inform future management of the condition, and which ones to take will therefore vary depending on the suspected cause of the collapse. For example, if the woman is haemorrhaging and this is the major cause of maternal collapse (RCOG 2011), blood tests should include full blood count (FBC), urea and electrolytes (U&Es), clotting screen and cross match of 6 units of blood.

Perimortem caesarean

Caesarean section should be considered primarily to aid the resuscitation of the mother, as her oxygen requirements will be less, venous return will be greater and cardiac compressions and ventilation will be more effective (RCOG 2011).

The 4-minute rule, from pulseless collapse to caesarean birth, originated from a case in which a mother who suffered cardiac arrest on the operating table was successfully resuscitated after the uterus was emptied (Katz et al 1986). However, this rule has been contested: following a systematic review of the evidence, Benson and colleagues (2016) concluded that to enhance the survival chances of both the mother and baby, the 4-minute rule should be replaced by 'immediately' (p. 256) once a decision to deliver the baby has been made.

Activity

Find out what equipment is needed for a perimortem caesarean. Where is it kept and where would such a procedure be performed?

Drug therapy

Drug therapy is secondary to effective CPR. There is debate about the effectiveness of drug therapy during cardiac arrest, and trials are ongoing to address this gap in the evidence. Until then, guidance is to administer adrenaline 1 milligram intravenously every 3 to 5 minutes (to raise blood pressure) followed by a bolus of 20 millilitres of 0.9% saline (British National Formulary 2018). Amiodarone 300 milligrams initially is considered after 3 shocks (to treat arrhythmia) (Resuscitation Council UK 2015).

Documentation

The use of a MEOWS chart should be ongoing. In addition, the contemporaneous documentation of all aspects of the process, from calling for help, commencing CPR, administering defibrillation etc. should be meticulously timed and recorded. After the event an incident form should be submitted to the risk/governance department so that the case can be reviewed and lessons learned to inform future clinical practice.

Debriefing

It is important that all people involved in the care of a woman who collapses have the opportunity to take part in a multi-professional debrief. Such an event should be to go through the sequence of events, what worked well and what could be improved. It should be about learning to enhance maternity care. Student midwives involved in providing care for the woman should also be involved and have the opportunity to ask questions and receive further support. It is good practice for the student's mentor to inform the university if a student was involved in a difficult or traumatic event, so that she can also receive support from her personal tutor.

Women and family members who experience maternal collapse may need expert help to understand what happened. This may require the input of clinical psychologists to avoid the development of or treat post-traumatic stress disorder or tokophobia, which is increasing after the rise in the incidence of severe maternal morbidity (Furuta et al 2012).

Conclusion

Maternal collapse can occur for a range of reasons; however, the principles of ensuring help is on the way, followed by opening the airway and starting CPR where indicated, are universal to its treatment. The midwife must start these emergency measures while help is on its way, and begin her assessment of the possible causes in parallel.

Resources
A guide to automated external defibrillators
https://www.resus.org.uk/publications/a-guide-to-aeds/
Pre-hospital resuscitation
https://www.resus.org.uk/resuscitation-guidelines/prehospital-resuscitation/
Adult basic life support
https://www.resus.org.uk/resuscitation-guidelines/adult-basic-life-support-and
-automated-external-defibrillation/
In hospital resuscitation
https://www.resus.org.uk/resuscitation-guidelines/in-hospital-resuscitation/
Left lateral uterine displacement
Zelop, C., Einav, S., Mhyre, J., Martin, S., 2017. Cardiac arrest during pregnancy: ongoing clinical conundrum. Am. J. Obstet. Gynecol. Doi: 10.1016/j.ajog.2017.12.232. p. 4.

References
Benson, M., Padovano, A., Bourjeily, G., Zhou, Y., 2016. Maternal collapse: challenging the four-minute rule. EBioMedicine 6, 253–257.

British National Formulary (BNF), 2018a. Adrenaline/epinephrine. Available at: https://bnf.nice.org.uk/drug/adrenalineepinephrine.html.

British National Formulary (BNF), 2018b. Amiodarone. Available at: https://bnf.nice.org.uk/drug/amiodarone-hydrochloride.html.

Coldridge, L., Davies, S., 2017. "Am I too emotional for this job?" An exploration of student midwives' experiences of coping with traumatic events in the labour ward. Midwifery 45, 1–6.

Davies, S., Coldridge, L., 2015. 'No man's land': an exploration of the traumatic experiences of student midwives in practice. Midwifery 31, 858–864.

Department of Health, 1993. Changing Childbirth: Report of the Expert Maternity Group Pt. II, Report of the Expert Maternity Group Pt.1. Department of Health, London.

Department of Health, 2004. National Service Framework for Children, Young People and Maternity Services. Standard 11. Maternity Services, Department of Health, London.

Department of Health, 2007. Maternity Matters: Choice, Access and Continuity of Care in a Safe Service. Department of Health, London.

Furuta, M., Sandall, J., Bick, D., 2012. A systematic review of the relationship between severe maternal morbidity and post-traumatic stress disorder. BMC Pregnancy Childbirth 12, 125.

Katz, V., Dotters, D., Droegemueller, W., 1986. Perimortem caesarean delivery. Obstet. Gynecol. 68, 571–576.

Kennedy, H., Doig, E., Hackley, B., et al., 2012. "The midwifery two-step": a study on evidence-based midwifery practice. J. Midwifery Womens Health 57, 454–460.

Knight, M., Nair, M., Tuffnell, D., et al. on behalf of MBRRACE-UK, 2017. Saving Lives, Improving Mothers' Care: Lessons Learned to Inform Maternity Care From the UK and Ireland Confidential Enquiries Into Maternal Deaths and Morbidity 2013–15. National Perinatal Epidemiology Unit, University of Oxford, Oxford.

Long, L., Penna, L., 2018. Maternal collapse. Obstet. Gynaecol. Reprod. Med. 28, 46–52.

National Maternity Review, 2016. Better births. Improving outcomes of maternity services in England. Available at: https://www.england.nhs.uk/wp…/national-maternity-review-report.pdf.

Nursing and Midwifery Council (NMC), 2009. Standards for Pre-Registration Midwifery Education. Nursing and Midwifery Council, London.

Nursing and Midwifery Council (NMC), 2015. The code: professional standards of practice and behaviour for nurses and midwives. Available at: https://www.nmc.org.uk/globalassets/sitedocuments/nmc-publications/nmc-code.pdf.

Resuscitation Council (UK), 2015. Adult basic life support and automated external defibrillation. adult-basic-life-support-and-automated-external-defibrillation.

Royal College of Obstetricians and Gynaecologists (RCOG), 2011. Maternal collapse in pregnancy and the puerperium. Green-top Guideline No.56. Available at: https://www.rcog.org.uk/globalassets/documents/guidelines/gtg_56.pdf.

Singh, S., McGlennan, A., England, A., et al., 2012. A validation study of the CEMACH recommended modified early obstetric warning system (MEOWS)*. Anaesthesia 67 (1), 12–18.

Smith, A., Edwards, S., Siassakos, D., 2012. Effective team training to improve outcomes in maternal collapse and perimortem caesarean section. Resuscitation 83, 1183–1184.

Zelop, C., Einav, S., Mhyre, J., Martin, S., 2017. Cardiac arrest during pregnancy: ongoing clinical conundrum. Am. J. Obstet. Gynecol. doi:10.1016/j.ajog.2017.12.232.

CHAPTER 2

Antepartum haemorrhage

TRIGGER SCENARIO

Elaine is 37 weeks into her pregnancy and suddenly feels a rush of warm fluid between her legs. When she investigates in the bathroom she realizes it is blood. She calls the hospital birth unit immediately and asks the midwife, Simone, on the end of the phone what she should do.

Introduction

Antepartum haemorrhage (APH) is defined in the UK as bleeding from the vaginal tract after the 24th week of gestation and before the birth of the baby (Royal College of Obstetricians and Gynaecologists (RCOG) 2011a). This definition is based on the current age of legal viability of the fetus in the UK, yet there are current ethical debates about this because of a potential survival of some babies at lower gestational ages (RCOG 2014). Before 24 weeks, any vaginal haemorrhage is classified as a threatened miscarriage or threatened abortion. In other countries the definition may be different, owing to the different applications of law and status of the unborn fetus.

Activity

Find out about legal viability of the fetus for the United States, Canada and Australia.

For any woman in whom this occurs, the experience will be upsetting and frightening, no matter when or at what stage of pregnancy bleeding occurs and how little blood is seen to be lost. Midwifery care should include emotional and psychological support and reassurance for the woman and her family.

APH can be a serious life-threatening condition for the woman and baby and therefore should be taken seriously. The latest triennial Confidential Enquiry into Maternal Death in the UK identifies women who died as a result of placental abruption (bleeding after separation of a normally situated placenta) or placenta praevia (bleeding from an abnormally situated placenta), the major causes of antenatal haemorrhage (Knight & Paterson-Brown 2017).

Types of APH

The types of haemorrhage during pregnancy could be described as minor or major, and a midwife may take more rapid emergency action in the latter case. The midwife should, however, be alert to the fact that concealed bleeding could be taking place within the uterine cavity, with only a small amount escaping, or sometimes the bleeding could be completely hidden.

Incidental bleeding

Bleeding may occur in different areas of the genital tract where there may be lesions or trauma. These could be:

+ Infection such as candidiasis
+ Vulval or vaginal varices
+ Cervical or uterine polyp
+ Cervical erosion or ectropion
+ Carcinoma of the cervix
+ Trauma
+ Haematuria

Activity

Find out about the aforementioned conditions and how they may be identified and treated.

In about 10% of cases of bleeding the cause will not be identified (antepartum bleeding of unknown origin), though these pregnancies appear to lead to more preterm birth and induction of labour (Bhandari et al 2014). It should also be remembered that a 'show' prior to starting labour may also be heavily blood stained. It has been suggested that approximately 45% of APH is related to a 'show' or unknown reasons, 5% related to the aforementioned conditions and the other 50% are due to the major placental causes (Higgins 2003).

Placental abruption or 'accidental' bleeding

In this circumstance a normally situated placenta begins to separate from the uterine wall prematurely; the condition is called abruptio placentae or an abruption (see Fig. 2.1). Recent UK statistics suggest that this affects approximately 0.43% of all pregnancies (NHS Digital 2016). The biggest risk factor for abruption is previous abruption, which increases the risk

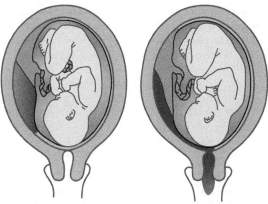

Fig. 2.1 Premature separation of the placenta (abruptio placentae). (With permission from Macdonald S, Johnson G, eds., Mayes midwifery, 15th ed., p. 906, Fig. 53.9)

Box 2.1 **Predisposing factors for placental abruption**

- Social deprivation
- Dietary deficiency such as inadequate folic acid or vitamin B_{12}
- Low body mass index (BMI)
- Male infant
- Hypertensive conditions
- Smoking
- Sudden decompression in the uterus
- Preterm prelabour rupture of membranes
- Previous history of placental abruption
- Illegal drug use
- Trauma, particularly abdominal
- Increasing maternal age
- Multiparity
- Fetal malposition
- Polyhydramnios
- Pregnancy after assisted reproductive techniques
- Intrauterine infection

(Combined from RCOG 2011a; Rosenberg et al 2011; Tikkanen 2011)

10-fold (Amokrane et al 2016). Sometimes this condition is referred to as *accidental*, but the circumstances are not always due to trauma and it may occur spontaneously for no known reason. There are, however, women who may be particularly at risk of placental abruption (see Box 2.1).

The reasons for placental abruption are multifactorial (Tikkanen 2011) and may also be connected to each other. For example, abruption of the placenta may lead to the risk of infection of the chorion, as likewise infection would potentially lead to the risk of an abruption. Smoking and hypertensive disease that lead to preterm birth may also be interrelated. Midwives should therefore be aware of these factors and be vigilant to the signs of bleeding.

Activity

Find out why smoking and hypertension may cause placental abruption.

What may cause sudden decompression in the uterus?

With this condition the bleeding may be obvious and revealed externally, concealed completely or partially revealed (see Fig. 2.2). It may also range in intensity from mild to severe, the latter of which will be a major emergency situation.

Activity

Find out what causes the bleeding to be revealed, concealed or partially revealed.

Prevention of placental abruption

It will not be possible to exclude completely the chance of abruption, as there are so many potential factors. Helping women to stop smoking or taking illegal drugs during pregnancy will have a beneficial effect, however, as well as potentially improving nutritional status (RCOG 2011a). Being aware of social deprivation and helping improve health to prevent preterm birth are important, as are encouraging women to wear seatbelts correctly when driving or riding in a car and awareness of potential situations of domestic abuse to help prevent abdominal trauma.

Diagnosis

If a woman has had a placental abruption, it may be difficult to identify if the bleeding is completely concealed. Bleeding may be obvious in approximately three-quarters of cases and accompanied by abdominal pain in about a third, which is usually continuous (RCOG 2011a). The cause of pain is unknown but may be related to stretching of the myometrium combined with blood being pushed back into the blood vessels. It is thought that a woman is less likely to experience abdominal pain if the placenta is attached to the posterior wall of the uterus; however, she could experience

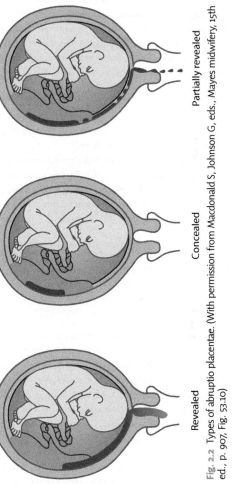

Revealed   Concealed   Partially revealed

Fig. 2.2 Types of abruptio placentae. (With permission from Macdonald S, Johnson G, eds., Mayes midwifery, 15th ed., p. 907, Fig. 53.10)

severe pain in her back or in her side. If a palpation is performed (which should be avoided if possible or carried out very gently and cautiously), the uterus may feel tense and rigid and larger than expected for the gestation of the pregnancy. It is sometimes described as 'couvelaire' or 'woody' (RCOG 2011a). The fetal parts will be difficult to palpate and there will probably be signs of fetal distress or death, as the fetus will have been deprived of oxygen and nutrients. The blood seen vaginally may be dark or 'old' blood. The woman will also be showing signs of shock, with an elevated pulse rate and low blood pressure. In severe cases the condition of the woman and her baby will deteriorate rapidly.

Placenta praevia or 'inevitable' bleeding

In this situation all or part of the placenta has implanted in the lower segment of the uterus, called placenta praevia, and could therefore be sited in front of the presenting part of the fetus.

The incidence of placenta praevia has been reported to be around 5.2 per 1000 pregnancies (Cresswell et al 2013). The most recent statistics in the UK suggest a figure of approximately 0.72% of births, which has increased in recent years. Types of placenta praevia have been classified into four categories (Hutcherson 2017; see Fig. 2.3).

Activity

Review the anatomy of the uterus and development of the placenta.
    Why would implantation in the lower segment increase the potential for bleeding?

Often the condition is categorized into two forms: minor if the placenta does not impinge on the cervical os and major if it covers or affects the os in any way (RCOG 2011b). An abnormal situation of the placenta may lead to serious outcomes, as reported in the most recent triennial Confidential Enquiries into Maternal Deaths, with nine women dying due to severe haemorrhage (Knight & Paterson-Brown on behalf of the haemorrhage and AFE chapter-writing group 2017).

The invasive placenta

Further serious situations occur when the placenta becomes morbidly adherent within the uterine cavity. The incidence of placenta accreta, increta and percreta, is approximately 1.7 per 10,000 births; however, this is vastly increased to 577 per 10,000 in situations in which women have had a previous caesarean section and placenta praevia (Fitzpatrick et al 2012). Where such a morbidly adherent placenta is identified antenatally, a specialist

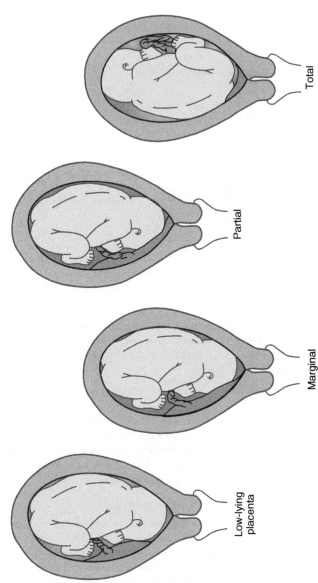

Fig. 2.3 Categories of placenta praevia. (With permission from Macdonald S, Johnson G, eds., Mayes midwifery, 15th ed., p. 904, Fig. 53.8)

multidisciplinary team will convene and radiological investigation including magnetic resonance imaging (MRI) will inform the management of the woman's care and decision on subsequent caesarean section (Kilcoyne et al 2017).

Activity

Find out what the following mean and check on the related anatomy:
- Placenta accreta
- Placenta increta
- Placenta percreta
- Vasa praevia

  Think about what the implications may be if you were caring for a woman with one of these conditions.

Detection of low-lying placenta

Identification of a low-lying placenta is often by means of an ultrasound scan in midpregnancy, but is felt to be over-reported at this stage. National Institute for Health and Care Excellence (NICE) guidance (2008, 2017) states that, as

> 'most low–lying placentas detected at the routine anomaly scan will have resolved by the time the baby is born, only a woman whose placenta extends over the internal cervical os should be offered another trans-abdominal scan at 32 weeks.'

A further transvaginal scan may be offered should this scan be inconclusive.

It is thought bleeding will occur when the lower uterine segments begin to increase in length with associated effacement of the cervix. Therefore the first episodes of bleeding may occur after 36 weeks' gestation. As with placental abruption, certain women are thought to be more at risk of the placenta implanting in the lower segment (see Box 2.2).

Prevention of an abnormal situation of a placenta

It is unlikely that the placenta embedding in an abnormal situation can be prevented in all cases. Avoiding caesarean section and other surgery on the uterus in previous pregnancies, unless completely necessary, would be one means of doing this. The main preventive measure would be supporting women in efforts to stop smoking as early as possible, or preferably preconception.

Box 2.2 **Predisposing factors for an abnormal condition of the placenta**

- Previous caesarean section
- Multiparity
- Increased maternal age
- Smoking
- Multiple pregnancy
- Increased placental size
- Previous induced abortion
- Previous myomectomy or hysterotomy
- Placental abnormality
- Pregnancy after assisted reproductive techniques

(Combined from Fitzpatrick et al 2012; Shobeiri & Jenabi 2017)

Activity

Consider why it would be appropriate to prevent women from being anaemic during pregnancy in relation to this condition.

Find out what advice is given about preventing anaemia in your locality.

Diagnosis

With the widespread use of ultrasound scanning, women and midwives may now be aware early of those at risk of bleeding from placenta praevia. It cannot, however, be excluded as a cause of bleeding after 20 weeks' gestation for those who may not have received antenatal care or have declined ultrasound scans. The bleeding may have started as a result of sexual intercourse and the woman will experience no pain. The blood may be bright red. On gentle palpation the uterus will usually feel relaxed, unless there are contractions in labour. The presenting part of the fetus may feel high or in an abnormal position, as the placenta will be lower in the uterus, preventing the fetus from moving down. Generally, the heart rate of the fetus will appear within normal ranges initially (RCOG 2011b).

Definitive diagnosis will be through ultrasound, and the use of trans-vaginal ultrasound is a safe option (RCOG 2011b).

APH – Management of care

If at any point during the care of a woman with APH, the woman's condition deteriorates and she requires resuscitation, the principles of managing maternal collapse, outlined in Chapter 1, should be followed.

In all cases of fresh vaginal bleeding in pregnancy, the midwife must provide psychological support and reassurance for the woman, who will be feeling very frightened and maybe very unwell. Medical assistance must be sought immediately, as this is potentially a life-threatening situation. In the community setting the assistance of paramedics should be summoned as a matter of course to enable transfer to the appropriate maternity unit.

The main aim of the initial care will be to assess and stabilize the woman's condition as quickly as possible and to establish the cause of the haemorrhage. If she has not had an ultrasound scan during early pregnancy placenta praevia should be considered as a potential cause. At no time should a vaginal examination be attempted. The following are actions a midwife may take:

- Position the woman on her side.
- Record temperature, pulse rate and blood pressure.
- Assess the fetal condition.
- Assess blood loss and change sanitary pads as necessary.
- Save soiled pads and clothes for blood estimation.
- Set up an intravenous infusion if there is significant blood loss.
- Give oxygen via a face mask.
- Continue frequent observations and document all results and actions until help arrives. (Hutcherson 2017)

Activity

- Read the emergency procedure for antepartum haemorrhage in the areas where you are located.
- Find out what intravenous fluids are used as first-line treatment.
- What is the procedure for obtaining blood products where you work?
- How do you care for a woman with a blood transfusion?

Depending on the seriousness of the maternal or fetal condition, medical management will include:

- The siting of an intravenous infusion with a large-bore cannula (if not already done), or possibly two
- Blood taken for group and cross-match for four units of blood, with close liaison with the haematologist on duty and the blood bank
- Full blood count, urea and electrolytes, clotting studies, fibrin degradation products and liver function tests
- Passing a Foley urinary catheter to monitor urine output
- Assessment for emergency birth of the fetus

(Hutcherson 2017; RCOG 2011a)

Assessment for the emergency birth of the fetus will depend on the number of factors related to the condition of the mother and the fetus and the cause of the bleeding. With placenta praevia bleeding may subside, which will result in a more stable situation. The woman may then be advised to stay as an inpatient within the unit for some time or until the birth of the baby. These women require particular psychological support, as they may experience feelings of isolation and loss of control (Katz 2001). In the majority of circumstances women may be cared for on an outpatient basis (RCOG 2011b).

In many cases women will need to be prepared for a caesarean section. There is insufficient evidence as to which form of anaesthetic is appropriate for women in this situation, and the anaesthetist will decide according to the individual circumstance (RCOG 2011b).

Complications

The potential problems associated with APH are related to the amount of blood lost and the effect on the woman and the unborn infant. The midwife should be aware of the following:

+ Blood coagulation disorders
+ Acute renal failure
+ Sheehan's syndrome
+ Postpartum haemorrhage
+ Infection
+ Anaemia
+ Psychological reactions

(Hutcherson 2017)

Activity

- Find out why the aforementioned conditions may occur after an antenatal bleeding episode.
- Find out about Sheehan's syndrome.
- What is disseminated intravascular coagulation?

The caregivers

It should also be remembered that any emergency situation will also be stressful for any family members present and for the professional carers concerned. Mechanisms should be in place to ensure that there is opportunity to debrief any concerns or questions about the care in a supportive and nonthreatening environment.

REFLECTION ON THE TRIGGER SCENARIO

Look back at the trigger scenario:

Elaine is 37 weeks into her pregnancy and suddenly feels a rush of warm fluid between her legs. When she investigates in the bathroom she realizes it is blood. She calls the hospital birth unit immediately and asks the midwife, Simone, at the end of the phone what she should do.

Now that you are familiar with bleeding in pregnancy, you should have some insight into the evidence and how the scenario relates to it. The jigsaw model will be used to explore the scenario in more depth:

Effective communication

Appropriate and effective communication is expected as an important part of a midwife's role (NMC 2015). This will include communication with the woman and her family as well as appropriate referral to other members of the multiprofessional team. In this scenario the midwife, Simone, needs to employ effective listening skills and ask important questions to establish what level of action should be taken. Questions that could be asked are: Is there a decision aid to inform the conversation? Where will Simone record the responses Elaine provides? What are the key responses she will give to Elaine? Who will Simone inform about this situation? How will she inform them?

Woman-centred care

It is expected that a woman should be central to her care and that she should have an informed choice around the decisions related to her care (National Maternity Review 2016). In an emergency situation, however, a woman may transfer this to the health professionals caring for her (Wang et al 2016). Questions that could be asked are: How can Simone provide information on the telephone that demonstrates compassion and respect while conveying the importance of receiving immediate care? How will Simone ensure she is concentrating on Elaine's story? What are the key things she will need to find out? What are the key questions she will ask? Why will she ask them?

Using best evidence

In this circumstance it is important to be aware of what the best evidence is surrounding the care of women with bleeding in pregnancy. Questions that could be asked are: Is the timing of the bleeding significant? Is this a complicated care circumstance? What are the possible causes for this bleeding? What is the evidence related to place of birth for women with previous APH? How would her labour be monitored where you work? Is there any evidence regarding conservative management versus immediate delivery in terms of maternal and neonatal outcomes?

Professional and legal issues

At all times the midwife should act professionally and according to the law. In relation to taking telephone calls and speaking to clients, she must act within her scope of practice (NMC). Questions that could be asked are: When using a telephone as part of Simone's professional role, are there any concerns regarding data protection? How will she maintain confidentiality yet share information with the multidisciplinary team? What are the expectations regarding recording the conversation? Should Simone be providing 'advice' or 'information'? If Simone gives 'advice' and Elaine chooses to ignore this, what are the implications? What is the law regarding Elaine's choices regarding her care? As the midwife answering the telephone, will Simone have responsibilities regarding what happens next?

Team working

In most situations in midwifery practice midwives do not work in isolation but are part of a wider multidisciplinary team. Within a hospital birth unit a midwife will be working with a team of colleagues. Questions that could be asked are: Who are the members of the multidisciplinary team who might contribute to Elaine's care? Who needs to know about Elaine's story first? Why, and what is their role? In what circumstance will Simone need to extend information about Elaine to another professional? Why should she tell him or her and how will she do this? In this complex circumstance, who is responsible for Elaine's care?

Clinical dexterity

In this situation related to a telephone call it is unlikely a midwife will require particular clinical dexterity. Should Elaine be asked to come into the unit, however, the midwife will need to be aware of her clinical needs. Questions that could be asked are: In this scenario what are Simone's clinical responsibilities? What observations should be carried out on Elaine when she arrives at the unit? What physical aspects of the examination should be carried out by Simone? What clinical examinations are contraindicated in these circumstances?

Models of care

There are a number of models of care practised across different areas with respect of complex needs. Questions that may be asked are: In this situation is Simone working within a centralized area as a triage midwife or as part of the team? Has she met Elaine before? Is she now going to be responsible for the care of Elaine should she be admitted to the unit, and therefore provide continuity? If not, will she be passing on information to someone else? What is the best model of care for a woman with complex needs?

Safe environment

At all times consideration should be made of the most appropriate environment for care of the woman and her baby. To establish the most appropriate environment of care the midwife has a responsibility to find out the relevant information to make decisions. If the woman is to be admitted to the maternity unit the environment should be prepared for her arrival. Questions that may be asked are: Where is the safest environment for Elaine's care? How will Simone establish the safest environment for Elaine? If Elaine needs urgent assistance, who should the midwife contact? Should Elaine drive to the hospital or does she require assistance, and by whom? How will Simone prepare the environment for Elaine for her safety?

Promotes health

The aim of all care is to promote the well-being of the woman and her baby. This will include her emotional, spiritual and social health as well as her physical needs. Questions that may be asked are: How may Simone promote Elaine's well-being during the telephone call? How may she help alleviate any anxieties she may have? How will Simone promote Elaine's well-being and that of her unborn baby if she is admitted to the unit? How will the midwife encourage Elaine to seek help again, if on this occasion she is discharged back to the community?

Further scenarios

SCENARIO 1

Colleen is 20 weeks pregnant with her second baby and attending the maternity unit for an ultrasound scan. While she is there she explains to the radiographer that she has been experiencing some occasional vaginal bleeding and has been feeling quite itchy 'down below'. The radiographer asks the clinic midwife to talk to her.

At any stage during pregnancy a woman may reveal that she has experienced some vaginal bleeding. If she mentions this, it is important the reason for the bleeding is established, and for any anxieties to be listened to as a priority. The radiographer here has therefore taken the appropriate steps for the cause to be investigated. At this stage of the pregnancy the ultrasound will have established the well-being of the fetus and the location of the placenta.

Further questions relevant to the scenario are:
+ What will the midwife establish from the radiographer about the ultrasound scan of the fetus and the placenta?
+ What questions will the midwife ask about the history of Colleen's pregnancy?
+ What questions will she ask about the current history of vaginal bleeding?
+ What investigations may need to be carried out to establish the cause of the bleeding?
+ Is the midwife trained to carry out these investigations or does she need to refer to anyone else?
+ What is the likely cause of bleeding at this stage of pregnancy?

SCENARIO 2

Cathy is admitted to the acute labour area by ambulance with a slight blood loss and severe, constant abdominal pain. She is 34 weeks pregnant and has a recent bruise on her abdomen. She informs Marian, the receiving midwife, that she fell down the stairs at home earlier in the day; however, there are no other fresh bruises to see.

It is important that the midwife is able to take a comprehensive history of the reason for Cathy's 'fall'. She needs to rule out a sudden loss of consciousness, a reason why she might have slipped or if the clinical presentation is consistent with a fall that is likely to have caused other bruising to outstretched arms or legs. Domestic violence is known to increase during pregnancy.

Further questions that could be asked are:
+ Has Cathy been asked during her pregnancy if she has ever felt threatened or feared for her safety?
+ Where and how often should this be asked and documented?
+ What systems are available and in operation where you work to alert the attending midwife that a woman may be a victim of domestic abuse?

+ What is the potential cause of Cathy's abdominal pain?
+ What clinical observations should Marian perform without delay?
+ Which members of the multidisciplinary team should be contacted immediately?

Conclusion

Bleeding during pregnancy may be an uncomplicated circumstance or a serious and catastrophic event. It is vital for the midwife to be aware of the potential for an emergency situation at all times and to be able to diagnose when this is taking place while recognizing it may be rare. Being aware of those particular women who may be more at risk will enable midwives to react swiftly when the situation does occur. Effective communication among all the carers is vital to ensure that the woman and her baby receive the safest possible care. At the same time, midwives have a particular role in providing psychological support to the woman and her family at a very stressful time. Preparation and practice of skills in this circumstance are essential in order for the multidisciplinary team to be ready for situations in which antenatal bleeding gives rise to maternal and fetal collapse.

Resources
RCOG Green Top Guidelines
Royal College of Obstetricians and Gynaecologists (RCOG). 2011a. Antepartum haemorrhage Green top guideline No. 63 https://www.rcog.org.uk/globalassets/documents/guidelines/gtg_63.pdf
Royal College of Obstetricians and Gynaecologists (RCOG). 2011b. Placenta Praevia, Placenta Praevia Accreta and Vasa Praevia: Diagnosis and Management Green Top guideline No: 27 https://www.rcog.org.uk/globalassets/documents/guidelines/gtg_27.pdf
Tommy's Charity Information for Women
https://www.tommys.org/pregnancy-information/pregnancy-complications/low-lying-placenta-placenta-praevia
https://www.tommys.org/pregnancy-information/pregnancy-complications/information-about-placental-abruption

References
Amokrane, N., Waterfield, A., Datta, S., Allen, E.R.F., 2016. Antepartum haemorrhage. Obstet. Gynaecol. Reprod. Med. 26 (2), 33–37.
Bhandari, S., Raja, E.A., Shetty, A., Bhattacharya, S., 2014. Maternal and perinatal consequences of antepartum haemorrhage of unknown origin. BJOG 12144–12152.
Cresswell, J.A., Ronsmans, C., Calvert, C., Filippi, V., 2013. Prevalence of placenta praevia by world region: a systematic review and meta-analysis. Trop. Med. Int. Health 18, 712–724.

Fitzpatrick, K.E., Sellers, S., Spark, P., et al., 2012. Incidence and risk factors for placenta accreta/increta/percreta in the UK: a national case-control study. PLoS ONE 7 (12), e52893.

Higgins, S., 2003. Obstetric haemorrhage. Emergen. Med. 15 (3), 227–231.

Hutcherson, A., 2017. Bleeding in pregnancy. In: MacDonald, S., Johnson, G. (Eds.), Mayes Midwifery, 15th ed. Elsevier, Oxford.

Katz, A., 2001. Waiting for something to happen: hospitalization with placenta previa. Birth 28 (3), 186–191.

Kilcoyne, A., Shenoy-Bhangle, A., Roberts, D., et al., 2017. MRI of placenta accreta, placenta increta, and placenta percreta: pearls and pitfalls. AJR Am. J. Roentgenol. 208 (1), 214–221.

Knight, M., Paterson-Brown, S., on behalf of the haemorrhage and AFE chapter-writing group. 2017. Messages for care of women with haemorrhage or amniotic fluid embolism. In: Knight M et al. (Eds.), Saving Lives, Improving Mothers' Care: Lessons Learned to Inform Maternity Care from the UK and Ireland. Confidential Enquiries into Maternal Deaths and Morbidity 2013–15. Available at: https://www.npeu.ox.ac.uk/downloads/files/mbrrace-uk/reports/MBRRACE-UK%20 Maternal%20Report%202017%20-%20Web.pdf.

National Maternity Review. 2016. Better births. Improving outcomes of maternity services in England. Available at: https://www.england.nhs.uk/wp-content/uploads/2016/02/national-maternity-review-report.pdf.

National Institute for Health and Care Excellence (NICE). 2008, 2017. Antenatal Care for uncomplicated pregnancies clinical guideline. Available at: https://www.nice.org.uk/guidance/cg62.

NHS Digital. 2016. NHS Maternity Statistics 2016–17. Available at: https://digital.nhs.uk/catalogue/PUB30137.

Nursing and Midwifery Council (NMC), 2015. The Code for Nurses and Midwives. NMC, London.

Rosenberg, T., Pariente, G., Sergienko, R., et al., 2011. Critical analysis of risk factors and outcome of placenta previa. Arch. Gynecol. Obstet. 284, 47.

Royal College of Obstetricians and Gynaecologists (RCOG). 2011a. Antepartum haemorrhage Green top guideline No. 63. Available at: https://www.rcog.org.uk/globalassets/documents/guidelines/gtg_63.pdf.

Royal College of Obstetricians and Gynaecologists (RCOG). 2011b. Placenta praevia, placenta praevia accreta and vasa praevia: diagnosis and Management Green Top guideline No. 27. Available at: https://www.rcog.org.uk/globalassets/documents/guidelines/gtg_27.pdf.

Royal College of Obstetricians and Gynaecologists (RCOG). 2014. Perinatal management of pregnant women at the threshold of infant viability (the obstetric perspective). Available at: https://www.rcog.org.uk/globalassets/documents/guidelines/scientific-impact-papers/sip_41.pdf.

Shobeiri, F., Jenabi, E., 2017. Smoking and placenta previa: a meta-analysis. J. Matern. Fetal Neonatal Med. 30 (24), 2985–2990.

Tikkanen, M., 2011. Placental abruption: epidemiology, risk factors and consequences. Acta Obstet. Gynecol. Scand. 90, 140–149.

Wang, L.H., Goopy, S., Lin, C.C., et al., 2016. The emergency patient's participation in medical decision-making. J. Clin. Nurs. 25, 2550–2558.

CHAPTER 3

Neonatal resuscitation

TRIGGER SCENARIO

Daniel was born and put straight into his mother's arms. His face was blue and he did not cry. With a look of panic on his face, his father asked, 'I thought they always cried?'

Introduction

Most babies are born capable of making the transition to extrauterine life without any assistance. However, some babies require intervention to help them initiate respiratory effort. Few require the additional support of cardiopulmonary resuscitation. These resuscitation guidelines are based on those produced by the Resuscitation Council (UK) in 2015; it is always a good idea to consult the Resuscitation Council (RCUK) website for updates, as guidance is refreshed when new evidence and best practice emerges.

Baby at risk

If there is reason to suspect that the baby may be born requiring some form of resuscitation, the resuscitation equipment should be checked, and if in a maternity unit, a paediatrician or neonatal nurse practitioner (NNP) should be called before the birth and introduced to the parents. His or her role and potential actions after the birth should be briefly explained to them. The overhead heater on the resuscitaire should be turned on and the platform positioned as close to the woman as possible to enable her to see her baby at all times. The paediatrician/NNP will quickly assess the baby for colour, tone, breathing and heart rate while the baby is with its mother. It is recommended that in preterm and uncompromised babies the cord should remain unclamped for at least 1 minute (Resuscitation Council 2015). Depending on the situation and apparent condition of the baby, it may be necessary to take the baby immediately to a resuscitaire to undertake a detailed assessment and initiate resuscitation without delay.

Activity

- In what circumstances should a midwife call a paediatrician/NNP to attend a birth?
- Whose responsibility is it to ensure the emergency equipment is checked where you work?

Unexpected need for resuscitation

Despite a complication-free labour, some babies do not breathe at birth. For this reason it is essential that cardiopulmonary resuscitation skills are practised regularly by attending specialist workshops for care of the neonate at birth. Guidance and equipment are subject to change as new technologies are developed and new research evidence informs practice. It is every midwife's duty to 'maintain the knowledge and skills you need for safe and effective practice' (Nursing and Midwifery Council 2015: 6.2).

Although it is not immediately apparent if some babies are going to breathe spontaneously and become pink and vigorous, it is immediately evident when a baby is born pale and floppy that further attention is required. A well baby may be born blue but should have a heart rate of more than 100 beats per minute, rising to the normal rate of 120 to 160 beats per minute (Solevag et al 2016). The baby will usually begin breathing within the first minute and then rapidly become pink (although its hands and feet may remain blue for some hours). A well baby will have a flexed tone and be moving all of its limbs.

Physiology of hypoxia

A fetus exposed to sustained hypoxia in utero or as it passes through the birth canal will need support to make the transition to extrauterine life (see Table 3.1). The outcome will depend on the degree and severity of this impaired oxygen supply as well as the gestation and resilience of the fetus. The sooner the hypoxia is interrupted the sooner the cascade of potential consequences can be halted (see Table 3.2).

Assessment of neonatal condition at birth

The first and most important action that should be taken is to dry the baby and replace damp towels with warm, dry ones to avoid further heat loss. During this process the baby will be stimulated and may begin to make a respiratory effort. This drying time also gives the midwife the chance to assess the baby's colour, tone, respiratory effort and heart rate and to summon further assistance if required. The head and neck should be in a straight line to maintain a patent airway.

Table 3.1: **Physiology of acute hypoxia**

Situation	Impact
Hypoxia in utero or during passage through the birth canal	Baby attempts to breathe
Continued hypoxia	Baby loses consciousness
Lack of oxygen to neural centres in the brainstem	Primary apnoea = absent respiratory effort
Heart rate decreases	Reduced perfusion of vital organs
Release of lactic acid	Increased respiratory acidosis
Hypoxia continues	Agonal gasps at rate 12/min
Gasps fade	Secondary or terminal apnoea; no further spontaneous breathing
Worsening acidosis	Impaired cardiac function
Heart rate falls	Death (20 minutes in term baby)

Table 3.2: **Resolution of hypoxia**

Situation	Action
Hypoxia in utero or during passage through the birth canal	Attendant ventilates the lungs
Oxygen from the lungs to the heart	Perfusion of the heart muscle
Heart rate increases	Neural centres in the brainstem perfused with oxygen
Neural centres in the brainstem regain normal function	Normal breathing and infant recovers

The heart rate can be assessed initially by placing two fingers over the centre of the baby's chest, while the stethoscope is being located and applied, for more accurate auscultation. If the baby's heart rate is less than 100 beats per minute and it is not making an effective respiratory effort, the cord should be securely clamped and cut to allow the baby to be moved to the resuscitaire or resuscitation area. The 1-minute Apgar score should be noted and the parents informed that you are taking the baby to the resuscitaire, as it needs some help to start breathing. Call for help.

Activity

- What is the Apgar score?
- When and how is it assessed?
- How do you call for help where you work?

Neonatal resuscitation

Where

Hospital labour wards are often designed for the benefit of the professionals who work there rather than for the new parents who frequent them. It would not be safe to try and resuscitate a baby on a high delivery bed in the middle of the room. The ventilation and suction equipment is usually attached to the wall or a resuscitaire and can be used only in a certain part of the room. Hence, in hospital it is usually imperative that resuscitation takes place away from the parents, but every effort should be made to keep the baby as close to its parents as possible. A running commentary should be made on the baby's progress, and the partner can also provide feedback to the mother.

If the woman is having a home birth, the ventilation and suction equipment should be checked and ready for immediate use in the unlikely event that they might be required. The room should be warm and draft free, and a supply of warm towels should be available. A safe place should be identified where resuscitation can take place, as this might not be immediately obvious if, for example, the woman is having a pool birth. If there is any suspicion that resuscitation may be required, paramedic help should be called immediately.

Temperature

Every effort should be made to ensure the baby is kept warm at a temperature between 36.5°C and 37.5°C (Resuscitation Council 2015). Hypothermic babies are less likely to respond to resuscitative measures and more likely to develop complications including hypoglycaemia, respiratory distress, pulmonary and intraventricular haemorrhage and sepsis (Chitty & Wyllie 2013).

Position of the neonate

The baby is placed on its back, on the resuscitaire, with its head facing downwards. The clock should be started and the overhead heater switched on. The oxygen supply should also be turned on. As with adult resuscitation, it is important to ensure that the airway is open. However, unlike in adult resuscitation, in the neonate this is achieved when its head is in the neutral position – that is, neither flexed forward nor extended backward. Because of the prominence of a newborn baby's occiput, which tends to make the head flex forward, the neutral position can be achieved by placing a towel under the baby's shoulders. It may be necessary to use a jaw thrust or chin lift manoeuvre if the baby has poor muscle tone.

Breathing

If the baby is not breathing its lungs will still be filled with fluid. If it has not made a successful respiratory effort by approximately 90 seconds, it will be necessary to administer five inflation breaths to disperse the fluid from the lungs. Inflation breaths are longer than ventilation breaths and require application of sustained pressure (about 30 cm of water) for 2 to 3 seconds (1–2–3; 2–2–3; 3–2–3; 4–2–3–; 5–2–3). The chest should rise with each breath. Air is administered to the baby via a bag and mask. The face mask for a baby is usually circular and made of soft silicone. It can be applied by holding it at the stem and rolling on from the base of the chin over the mouth and nose. It is then held over the baby's nose and mouth with the nondominant hand while the dominant hand squeezes the bulbous oxygen chamber. The heart rate should then be rechecked.

If the heart rate is increasing but the baby does not start to breathe, then ventilation breaths should be given via the face mask at a rate of 30 to 40 per minute, until the baby starts to breathe for itself.

If the heart rate does not increase then you need to ask:
+ Did the chest rise with the inflation breaths?
+ Is the airway open?
+ Is a jaw thrust required?
+ Is there an airway obstruction?

If after five effective inflation breaths the heart rate remains below 60 beats per minute and 30 seconds of ventilation breaths, then chest compressions should be commenced.

Chest compressions

If chest compressions are needed, help should be on its way and a pulse oximeter applied if available. Compressions should be started only once the lungs have been successfully aerated. The purpose of chest compressions is to compress the heart between the sternum and the backbone so that blood is forced from the heart into the circulation (Solevag et al 2016).

The quality of chest compressions is multifaceted and determined by a combination of rate, compression to ventilation ratio and the force applied (Solevag & Schmolzer 2017):

1. Rate: 90/minute
2. Ratio: 3 compressions to 1 ventilation
3. Reduce the anterior–posterior chest diameter by one-third

Chest compressions are best performed on a baby by gripping the chest with both hands so that the thumbs of both hands are positioned on the sternum just below the line of the nipples. The fingers are positioned on the baby's back over its spine. The chest should be compressed so as to reduce its height by approximately one-third, and a quick, firm action should be used. There should be three compressions for each inflation of the lungs, and an increased oxygen concentration should be considered (Resuscitation Council 2015).

Paediatric care

When the paediatrician arrives, she or he may wish to intubate the baby, depending on its response to bag-and-mask ventilation. It will be helpful to assist the paediatrician by anticipating her or his need for appropriate equipment. The paediatrician will also need information about the birth and how the baby has or has not responded to resuscitation so far. The Apgar score should be assessed again after 5 minutes and, if below 7, again after 10 minutes.

Drugs

If the baby does not respond to cardiopulmonary resuscitation (there is no significant cardiac output), it may be necessary for the paediatrician to administer drugs. This is usually achieved via the umbilical vein using a catheter. The three drugs that may be used are:

- Adrenaline (0.1 ml/kg of a 1:10 000 solution)
- Sodium bicarbonate (2–4 ml of 4.2% bicarbonate solution)
- Glucose (2.5 ml/kg of 10% glucose).

Activity
- When should vitamin K be administered intramuscularly?
- What is the rationale for giving vitamin K to a baby who requires resuscitation?

Further treatment

If the baby has required more than brief intermittent positive pressure ventilation (IPPV) by face mask, it will need further observation in a special care environment. The baby should have name labels (previously checked with the parents) securely attached to both ankles before it leaves the labour room. The parents should be kept fully informed of the baby's condition and should be encouraged to visit as often as they are able.

Activity

Consider how the midwife can address the emotional needs of parents whose baby requires resuscitation at birth.

Meconium-stained amniotic fluid

The incidence of the fetus passing meconium in utero increases with maturity and is rare at less than 37 weeks' gestation. The incidence of meconium-stained amniotic fluid (MSAF) is about 20% to 30% at term, increasing to up to 52% at 42 weeks' gestation (Argyridis & Arulkumaran 2016). If there is meconium-stained liquor, it is common hospital practice to call a paediatrician/NNP to attend the birth. If the baby inhales meconium then it is at risk of developing meconium aspiration syndrome (MAS), a rare but potentially fatal complication.

It was once considered good practice to perform oropharyngeal and nasopharyngeal suctioning on the baby before the shoulders emerged; however, this is no longer the case (Resuscitation Council 2015). In a multicentre, randomized controlled trial (Vain et al 2004), 2514 women with MSAF were randomized for their babies to receive suctioning of the oropharynx followed by suctioning of the nasopharynx or no suction. There were no differences between the treatment and control groups for the incidence of MAS, need for or duration of mechanical ventilation, mortality, oxygen therapy or hospital care.

Oropharynx suctioning should be considered and performed only under direct visualization in the presence of 'thick, viscous meconium in a non-vigourous infant' (Resuscitation Council 2015).

Activity

- What is the incidence of meconium-stained liquor at term?
- What is the incidence of meconium aspiration syndrome?
- What are the complications of oesophageal suction in neonates?
- What is the treatment for meconium aspiration syndrome?

Once the baby is born, if it breathes spontaneously, has a heart rate of more than 100 beats per minute and has a good tone then no immediate action is necessary other than regular observations of temperature and respiration rate. Intubation of otherwise well babies can result in trauma to the baby and does not reduce the incidence of MAS or other respiratory conditions (Wiswell et al 2000).

Most hospital and home birth guidelines suggest that babies who passed meconium in utero should be observed in hospital for a time, so that their respiration rate can be monitored. Although this does not usually present a problem for babies born in hospital, for those born at home it involves considerable disruption to the family unit after an otherwise uncomplicated birth.

Activity

- Find out what the guidelines are where you work for monitoring babies who passed meconium in utero.
- Research the role of amnioinfusion for meconium-stained liquor in labour.

REFLECTION ON THE TRIGGER SCENARIO

Look back on the trigger scenario at the start of the chapter.

Daniel was born and put straight into his mother's arms. His face was blue and he did not cry. With a look of panic on his face, his father asked, 'I thought they always cried?'

The scenario is one that midwives can encounter without any prior warning but need to be able to manage in a calm and professional manner. Now that you are familiar with the principles of neonatal resuscitation, you will have insight into how the scenario relates to the evidence. The jigsaw model will now be used to explore the trigger scenario in more depth.

Effective communication

This scenario clearly presents as an alarming situation for new parents and potentially for inexperienced midwives. However, the midwife's demeanour and tone of voice can go a long way to help reassure parents that their child is in safe hands. Questions that arise from the scenario might include: How might the midwife have prepared the parents for how the baby might look or behave when first born? What might the midwife say to the father about the condition of his child? How can the midwife demonstrate through her body posture and tone of voice that she is competent to manage this situation?

Woman-centred care

Throughout pregnancy and the baby's birth, the midwife has an important role to play in establishing the individual hopes and aspirations of women and what they wish for at the time of birth. She can therefore help the woman retain control of her situation by continuing to involve her in decisions and care of the baby at birth. Questions that arise from the scenario might include: Had the woman expressed a wish to have immediate skin-to-skin contact at birth? Had she been given information antenatally to help her make an informed decision about this? How can the parents be involved in the immediate efforts to stimulate the baby to breathe? How can the parents continue to be involved in the baby's progress if the baby needed resuscitation?

Using best evidence

We are required to use best evidence to support our decision making and care planning, wherever such evidence exists. It is therefore important that we keep up to date with recent local and national guidance to help inform our practice. Questions that arise from the scenario might include: How often are the UK resuscitation guidelines revised? What have been the major changes in recent times regarding the use of oxygen for ventilation purposes? Why is this the case? Why do we no longer use suction routinely on healthy newborn infants? What might have predisposed this infant to be reluctant to breath at birth? Think about a time when you observed a mentor practise in a way that you knew not to be evidence based. Did you ask her about it? Why?

Professional and legal issues

When an emergency situation arises, it is important that we capture the sequence of events accurately and as concurrently as possible. This can be difficult in a situation in which many different people may come to assist or the adrenaline is flowing. Questions that arise from the scenario might include: What tools are available to help you record the sequence of resuscitation in a timely manner? What training requirements are you required to comply with in regard to neonatal resuscitation? What is the role of revalidation in supporting you to learn from new and challenging situations? What is the role of the employer with regard to providing training opportunities in relation to your role as a midwife?

Team working

Providing swift and effective resuscitation requires that midwives work with neonatal colleagues to provide timely evidence-based care to all babies who require support to make the transition to the outside world. This multi-professional effort requires us to have a working knowledge of our role and limitations within it, so that we know when to call for help and what that help can provide. Questions that arise from the scenario might include: Is there multi-professional training for those who work together to learn together? Who might this include for optimum learning? What would the midwife do with Daniel before she called for team help? Which team is best placed to offer support to the parents? Which members of the team can provide support at a home birth?

Clinical dexterity

During a resuscitation it is important that the correct equipment is at hand and in working order. The midwife needs to know how it works and be able to use it. She needs to be confident to engage the parents in drying and stimulating Daniel, replacing damp towels and being ready to clamp and cut the cord if he does not start to breathe. Questions that arise from the scenario might include: Had the midwife checked that the resuscitaire was in full working order before Daniel was born? When did the midwife last practise using a bag and mask? Does she know how to insert an airway if needed to maintain a patent airway? Can she apply oximetry to the baby if needed to monitor oxygen saturation?

Models of care

If the midwife is working in a caseload model, it is likely that she will have previously met Daniel's parents and have established a trusting relationship built on mutual respect. However, if working in a traditional model of care in which midwives who work in the maternity unit do not work in the community, this is unlikely to be the case, and a relationship must be quickly developed during labour. Questions that arise from the scenario might include: How might the model of care influence the place of birth? If Daniel was born at home, what resources could the midwife draw on to provide effective resuscitation to Daniel? What are the advantages of continuity of care in this situation?

Safe environment

Any resuscitation situation can involve many professionals coming into the same room at the same time, and it has the potential to become chaotic if not carefully managed. There should be a lead professional who is directing the activities as well as someone documenting times and interventions as they happen. It is imperative that the professionals involved do not put themselves in danger, and reducing the risk of slips, trips and falls is part of the process. Questions that arise from the scenario might include: If the midwife had suspected fetal compromise during labour, what actions could be taken before the birth to be able to commence active resuscitation immediately? Where is the best place for the birth partner to be if the baby is taken to the resuscitaire? How is the risk of infection reduced during resuscitation? What safeguards are built into the resuscitaire to reduce the risk of overinflation of the lungs?

Promotes health

All clinical situations are an opportunity to provide a role model to new parents and show them safe techniques for providing baby care. Providing a running commentary on all care given is both reassuring to parents and a learning moment. For example, the midwife can encourage the parents to talk to Daniel, explaining that he will already recognize their voices. It can be explained that while he is in skin-to-skin contact with his mother her body heat will help keep him warm and that if he needs to go to the resuscitaire a heater will provide warmth until he can return to his parents. Questions that arise from the scenario might include: How can the partner be encouraged to support the mother's emotional well-being during this time? What can the midwife do to promote responsive care if Daniel needs to go to the neonatal unit?

Further scenarios

The following scenarios enable you to consider how specific situations influence the care the midwife provides. Use the jigsaw model to explore the issues raised in the scenario.

SCENARIO 1

Baby Amelia is born by emergency caesarean section after her mother had a placental abruption. The caesarean was performed under general anaesthetic, as the fetal heart was 80 beats per minute on admission.

Practice point

Caesarean birth is increasingly common; however, it is infrequently performed under general anaesthetic, more commonly under a spinal block. Baby Amelia is likely to require support to begin extrauterine life; the degree of intervention needed will depend on her gestation, growth and a range of other factors.

Questions that arise from the scenario might include:

+ What is the normal range for the fetal heart at term?
+ How long can the fetus compensate for a reduced oxygen supply?
+ How quickly can a woman be transferred to theatre from admission to labour ward, where you work?
+ What are the implications for the fetus of using a general anaesthetic?
+ Which professionals should be present at the birth to care for baby Amelia?
+ What are the first five actions to be taken when the baby is born with no respiratory effort?
+ Where is the birth partner and who is looking after him or her?

SCENARIO 2

Katy is being cared for on the Midwife Led Unit, which is not attached to the Consultant Unit 5 miles away. It is Katy's first baby and she is approaching the second stage of labour, having managed her pain with Entonox and support from her midwife, Sue. After the last contraction, Sue listens to the fetal heart, which is 100 beats per minute (bpm) initially and then recovers quickly to 120 bpm. Sue looks at Katy's pad and notices that the liquor now draining is slightly meconium stained.

Practice point

It is not uncommon for babies that are post-term to pass meconium before birth. However, the aspiration of meconium is known to be a serious situation for the neonate and one that can lead to significant morbidity.

Questions that arise from the scenario might include:

+ What gestation has Katy reached?
+ What are the criteria for transfer to a consultant unit in your locality?
+ How often should Sue be auscultating the fetal heart?
+ Is the current fetal heart rate reassuring?
+ What action should Sue take regarding her findings?
+ What action should be taken at the birth?
+ What observations are required on the baby postnatally?

Resources

Resuscitation of premature infants

Katheria, A., Poeltler, D., Durham, J., et al., 2016. Neonatal resuscitation with an intact cord: a randomized clinical trial. J. Pediatr. 178, 75–80.

Resuscitation training

Dempsey, E., Pammi, M., Ryan, A.C., Barrington, K.J., 2015. Standardised formal resuscitation training programmes for reducing mortality and morbidity

in newborn infants. Cochrane Database Syst. Rev. (9), CD009106, doi:10
.1002/14651858.CD009106.pub2.

Suction at birth

Foster, J.P., Dawson, J.A., Davis, P.G., Dahlen, H.G., 2017. Routine oro/
nasopharyngeal suction versus no suction at birth. Cochrane Database Syst.
Rev. (4), CD010332, doi:10.1002/14651858.CD010332.pub2.

MBRRACE 2017 perinatal confidential enquiry

Field, D., Wardle, S., Jones, T., Johnston, E. Resuscitation and neonatal care. In:
Term, Singleton, Intrapartum Stillbirth and Intrapartum-Related Neonatal Death.
Available at: https://www.npeu.ox.ac.uk/downloads/files/mbrrace-uk/reports/
MBRRACE-UK%20Intrapartum%20Confidential%20Enquiry%20Report%20
2017%20-%20final%20version.pdf.

References

Argyridis, S., Arulkumaran, S., 2016. Meconium stained amniotic fluid. Obstet.
Gynaecol. Reprod. Med. 26, 227–230.

Chitty, H., Wyllie, J., 2013. Importance of maintaining the newly born temperature
in the normal range from delivery to admission. Semin. Fetal Neonatal Med.
18, 362–368.

Nursing and Midwifery Council. 2015. The code: professional standards of practice
and behaviour for nurses and midwives. Available at: https://www.nmc.org.uk/
globalassets/sitedocuments/nmc-publications/nmc-code.pdf.

Resuscitation Council (UK). 2015. Resuscitation and support of transition of
babies at birth. Available at: https://www.resus.org.uk/resuscitation-guidelines/
resuscitation-and-support-of-transition-of-babies-at-birth/.

Solevåg, A., Cheung, P., O'Reilly, M., et al., 2016. A review of approaches to optimise
chest compressions in the resuscitation of asphyxiated newborns. Arch. Dis.
Child. Fetal Neonatal Ed. 101 (3), F272.

Solevag, A., Schmolzer, G., 2017. Optimal chest compression rate and compression
to ventilation ratio in delivery room resuscitation: evidence from newborn piglets
and neonatal manikins. Front Pediatr. 5, 3. doi:10.3389/fped.2017.00003.

Vain, N.E., Szyld, E.G., Prudent, L.M., et al., 2004. Oropharyngeal and nasopharyngeal suctioning of meconium-stained neonates before delivery of their shoulders:
multicenter, randomised controlled trial. Lancet 364, 597–602.

Wiswell, T., Gannon, C., Jacob, J., et al., 2000. Delivery room management of the
apparently vigorous meconium-stained neonate: results of the multicenter,
international collaborative trial. Pediatrics 105 (Pt 1), 1–7.

CHAPTER 4

Breech birth

TRIGGER SCENARIO

The ambulance man pushed Julie through the labour ward doors in a wheelchair. She was 37 weeks pregnant with her second baby and in established labour. 'I want to push!' she shouted. The midwife showed them into a labour room and helped Julie out of the chair. She leaned over the bed, pushing involuntarily. After that contraction Julie said, 'The last time I saw my midwife she thought he was breech.'

Introduction

Approximately 4% of babies present by the breech at term (Ferreira et al 2015), and the rate is higher in preterm pregnancies. There has been a marked decline in the proportion of breech babies born vaginally in recent years, which, in turn, has led to a decline in the expertise of both midwives and obstetricians who attend breech births. However, student midwives need to learn and practise the art of caring for women with a breech presentation in labour, as in some women it may be undiagnosed until labour starts. Qualified midwives also need regular updates and opportunities to maintain and develop their skills and practice. This chapter focuses on the management of a breech presentation in labour.

Activity

- What maternal and fetal factors predispose the baby to present by the breech?
- What is the proportion of breech presentation at 28 and 34 weeks' gestation?

The Term Breech Trial

In 2000 Hannah et al published the results of a randomized controlled trial designed to establish the safest way for term breech babies to be born. It involved 2088 women from 26 countries and concluded that planned caesarean section was safer for the baby than vaginal birth with a skilled attendant. There were no differences between the groups regarding serious maternal complications. This controversial conclusion has led to the widespread adoption of elective caesarean for breech babies, further reducing the experience and expertise of maternity care providers in breech birth care. Subsequent professional debate has led to many rejecting its conclusions, not least because of its inclusion criteria and how they conflict with a woman-centred, midwifery model (Fahy 2011). In a subsequent trial (Goffinet et al 2006) in which planned vaginal breech was usual practice, providing certain criteria were observed, there was no difference between the groups, and vaginal breech birth for singleton pregnancies was heralded as a safe option.

There should be no complacency regarding the fact that many breech babies are born by caesarean. Midwives need to be prepared to care for women who decline surgical delivery and therefore need the support of calm and competent practitioners to birth their baby with confidence. Midwives also need the skill to look after women who present for care in established labour with a breech presentation. It may be that a woman has planned to have an elective caesarean section for the birth of her baby, but she may present to the labour ward in the second stage of labour. When the breech is advancing and all the medical staff are in theatre, the midwife needs to know what to do.

Activity

Read the paper describing the Term Breech Trial (Hannah et al 2000). What are the limitations of this study and how could it have been improved?

Who provides care?

If a midwife diagnoses this mal-presentation, according to the Nursing and Midwifery Code (Nursing and Midwifery Council 2015), she is obliged to 'make a timely and appropriate referral to another practitioner when it is in the best interests of the individual needing any action, care or treatment' and 'ask for help from a suitably qualified and experienced healthcare professional to carry out any action or procedure that is beyond the limits of your competence' (NMC 2015: 15). Indeed the Royal College of Obstetricians and Gynaecologists (RCOG) Green-top Guideline (Impey et al 2017) recommends 'the presence of a skilled birth attendant is essential for safe vaginal breech birth.'

Although the care of the woman who has a baby who presents by the breech in labour will generally be overseen by a senior obstetrician, some doctors will enable the midwife to continue to provide care while they

Box 4.1 **Summary of rationale for midwives to be competent at breech birth care**

Midwives need to be competent to attend a breech birth when:
- Women want a vaginal breech birth
- Woman want a caesarean but go into labour before admission
- Women present for care in advanced labour with an undiagnosed breech presentation
- Medical attendant is not available

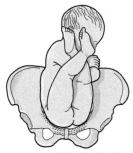

Fig. 4.1 Frank breech. (With permission from Marshall J, Raynor M, eds., Myles Textbook for Midwives, 16th ed., p. 359, Fig. 16.27. Edinburgh: Churchill Livingstone/Elsevier.)

provide support and guidance. Box 4.1 summarizes the rationale for midwives to be competent at breech birth care.

Types of breech presentation

The most common type of breech presentation is one in which the hips are flexed and the knees extended – known as a 'frank' breech (Fig. 4.1). Less common is the complete breech presentation, in which the knees and the hips of the fetus are flexed and the feet are above the buttocks (Fig. 4.2). Rarely the fetus presents with a foot, and this is known as a footling breech (Fig. 4.3). Occasionally the hip is extended and the knee is the presenting part (Fig. 4.4).

Diagnosing breech presentation antenatally

Where a breech presentation is diagnosed in pregnancy the woman should be offered external cephalic version (ECV). If this does not work or she declines, she should have access to skilled counselling and a personal risk assessment to enable her to make an informed decision about how the birth is managed. If she opts for a vaginal breech birth, she should be informed

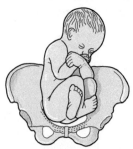

Fig. 4.2 Complete breech. (With permission from Marshall J, Raynor M, eds., Myles Textbook for Midwives, 16th ed., p. 359, Fig. 16.28. Edinburgh: Churchill Livingstone/Elsevier.)

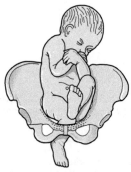

Fig. 4.3 Footling breech. (With permission from Marshall J, Raynor M, eds., Myles Textbook for Midwives, 16th ed., p. 359, Fig. 16.29. Edinburgh: Churchill Livingstone/Elsevier.)

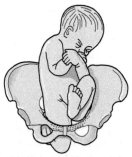

Fig. 4.4 Knee presentation. (With permission from Marshall J, Raynor M, eds., Myles Textbook for Midwives, 16th ed., p. 359, Fig. 16.30. Edinburgh: Churchill Livingstone/Elsevier.)

of the relative risks and a meticulously documented plan of care should be agreed with her and provision made for its implementation. If she chooses elective caesarean birth this should be arranged for 39 weeks' gestation and she should be informed of the increased risk to future pregnancies of repeat caesarean and abnormal placentation (Impey et al 2017).

Diagnosing breech presentation in labour

Detecting a breech presentation before labour requires the midwife to use all of her skills. However, if the woman has an elevated body mass index (BMI) this can sometimes make the palpation difficult, and when the baby splints its head with its feet, as in a frank breech, the head can feel like a bottom. Approximately 8% or more of breeches remain undetected until labour starts (Ressl & O'Beirne 2015).

History

Sometimes the history given by the woman alerts the midwife to suspect that the baby may be presenting by the breech – for example, if the woman complains of feeling particularly uncomfortable under her ribs (because of the location of the fetal head).

Abdominal palpation

An abdominal palpation should be performed to determine the presentation of the fetus, although this may be difficult to establish, especially if the legs are extended (Fig. 4.1). In a complete breech (Fig. 4.2) presentation, it may be possible to locate the fetal head at the fundus and ballot it independently of its back. When palpating the presenting part, the midwife may note that there is no indentation where she might expect the head to join the shoulders, as she palpates the continuous line of the fetal back. However, this finding might lead her to suspect that the fetal head is deeply engaged in the pelvis. The proportion of the baby that remains palpable abdominally should alert her to suspect that the baby is presenting by the breech.

Auscultation

The fetal heart is often heard loudest at or above the umbilicus when the baby presents by the breech. However, when the breech descends into the pelvis, the fetal heart may be heard below the umbilicus, as in a cephalic presentation.

Vaginal examination

It can be difficult to discern a breech presentation if the cervix is uneffaced or less than 3 centimetres dilated. The breech feels irregular, smooth (hair free) and soft, and care should be taken not to damage the soft tissues of the genitalia. No suture lines or fontanelles can be felt, and fresh meconium may be seen on the gloves if the membranes have ruptured. If a limb is detected it is essential to distinguish between the hand and the foot.

All of the foregoing observations should be considered together before the midwife concludes that the baby is presenting by the breech. The woman and her partner should be informed of her suspicions and the course of action that might follow. The woman should remain an active partner in decisions about her care and be given the opportunity to ask questions and consider the options available.

Activity

- What antenatal exercises are sometimes recommended to women with a breech presentation, and what is their value?
- What is external cephalic version (ECV)?
- When should ECV be attempted and when is it contraindicated?

It's a breech – what now?

Immediate actions

After a breech presentation is suspected, the midwife caring for the woman should inform the midwife who is coordinating the labour ward and also inform the medical staff. The presentation of the baby is often confirmed using ultrasound, and if there is enough time the position and estimated fetal weight should be ascertained. The presence of risk factors, the wishes of the mother and availability of a skilled birth attendant will contribute to the recommendations and decision about the management of care (Table 4.1). The theatre team should be alerted. If the woman is in the second

Table 4.1: **Informed decision making**

Caesarean recommended	Vaginal breech birth considered
Hyperextended neck on ultrasound	Maternal request
High estimated fetal weight (more than 3.8 kg)	Spontaneous onset of labour
Low estimated weight (less than tenth centile)	Term fetus
Footling presentation	No known fetal abnormality
Evidence of antenatal fetal compromise	Skilled attendants available
Prolonged first stage of labour	Normal labour progress

stage of labour, senior medical attendance should be requested, including paediatric support. However, RCOG guidance now states that 'Women near or in active second stage of labour should not be routinely offered caesarean section' (Impey et al 2017).

Undiagnosed breech at home

Before a planned home birth it is usual for the midwife to discuss with the woman situations that might require transfer to hospital. As such, the detection of a breech presentation during labour should be one that has already been discussed and a plan of action agreed on.

If an undiagnosed breech is detected in a woman planning a home birth and she is in the second stage of labour, judgement would need to be made regarding the most appropriate course of action. This would need to take account of the woman's wishes, her well-being and that of the baby, progress of the labour up to this point, parity and distance from the hospital. A paramedic ambulance should be summoned to avoid delay if transfer to hospital becomes necessary. Even if birth is not imminent, arrangements for transfer to hospital should be made and the receiving hospital forewarned so that the appropriate professionals are awaiting the woman's arrival.

Informed choice

As with the diagnosis of a breech presentation in the antenatal period, diagnosing a breech in labour will require that the midwife is able to develop and maintain a relationship with the mother to enable the free exchange of information and support. In line with professional guidance the midwife will: 'Encourage and empower people to share decisions about their treatment and care' and 'respect, support and document a person's right to accept or refuse care and treatment' (NMC 2015). These principles must be maintained throughout the birthing process.

Care during spontaneous breech birth

Maternal observations

It is important to remember the general principles of labour care during a breech birth. The woman should be consulted about all aspects of her care, informed of her progress, praised for her efforts and given lots of encouragement. Her blood pressure, temperature and pulse should be measured regularly and recorded on the partogram. The length, strength and frequency of her uterine contractions should also be observed and recorded.

It is important to confirm full dilatation of the cervix before encouraging active pushing by the woman. This is to avoid the potential complication of the breech passing through a partially dilated cervix and the after-coming head being trapped by it. Maternal effort should be encouraged only if the breech is visible (Impey et al 2017).

Monitoring of the fetal heart

The well-being of the fetus should also be monitored. The RCOG Green-top Guideline (Impey et al 2017) recommends continuous electronic fetal monitoring with consent. The fetal heart rate should be between 110 and 160 beats per minute and reactive to activity (National Institute for Health and Care Excellence 2014, 2016). Fetal buttock sampling is not recommended. Where there is any concern about the fetal heart before the second stage of labour, a caesarean should be considered.

Monitoring progress

When the fetus is at term and there are no apparent contraindications to spontaneous birth, the midwife should watch, wait and monitor progress but keep her hands to herself. 'Hands off the breech' is the old adage that has been the golden rule of successful breech birth. It is suspected that operators who attempt to interfere with the normal mechanism are the cause of poor neonatal outcomes.

With maternal effort the breech will distend the perineum, causing it to thin out.

All-fours position

There is some evidence based on expert opinion that birth on all fours (Fig. 4.5) results in spontaneous birth more readily than in the supine position and results in less trauma to the mother (Bogner et al 2015).

As with spontaneous vaginal birth, once the mechanism for breech birth is understood the principles can be applied to situations in which women adopt a range of positions. Learn and understand the mechanism for breech birth in both all-fours/standing and semi-recumbent; turn the book, the doll and pelvis or the mannequin upside down and work out how the breech will birth in these positions. For a detailed description of a breech birth with the woman on all fours, refer to Evans (2012).

Activity

- Consider your own view about vaginal breech birth and the factors that have influenced it.
- Is vaginal breech birth actively supported where you work?

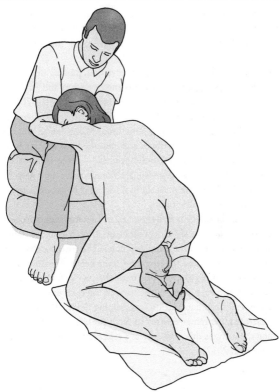

Fig. 4.5 Spontaneous breech birth. (With permission from Marshall J, Raynor M, eds., Myles Textbook for Midwives, 16th ed., p. 382, Fig. 17.8. Edinburgh: Churchill Livingstone/Elsevier.)

Mechanism of spontaneous breech birth

As this chapter is about how to care for women in a potential emergency situation, the description of the mechanism of breech birth that follows involves the woman in a supported semi-recumbent position and the foot and end of the bed removed, to enable the baby to be born and hang down and the practitioner have access to perform the required maneuvers.

Where practitioners are experienced and competent in facilitating breech birth on all-fours, women should be able to adopt the position that they feel most comfortable with. As most obstetricians are more familiar with performing an assisted breech birth with the mother in a dorsal position, she should be aware that she may be asked to turn over if such intervention is required, depending on the skill and experience of the attending practitioner.

The anterior hip of the baby usually emerges first, passing under the symphysis pubis. The posterior hip distends the perineum and emerges with lateral flexion, described as 'rumping' (Downe & Marshall 2014). External rotation takes place, with the fetal back uppermost (when the woman is in the dorsal position). The fetus should continue to emerge with maternal effort. Once the umbilicus emerges, the fetus continues to descend, and the legs will escape spontaneously – there is no need to manipulate them. The cord will be visible, although there is no need to touch it. At this point it will be possible to note the baby's tone (should be flexed) and colour (should be pink).

The elbows should be on the baby's chest and will emerge spontaneously with the next contraction. The shoulders rotate on the pelvic floor and the anterior shoulder escapes under the symphysis pubis. The posterior shoulder emerges from the perineum and the head enters the pelvis. The fetus then hangs unsupported to bring the occiput onto the pelvic floor, where it rotates forward. After a minute or so the nape of the neck emerges. The safe birth of the fetal head depends on it remaining flexed and emerging slowly. The midwife must remain poised to catch the baby at all times but avoid touching the baby, as this may initiate a reflex extension of the arms or head (Impey et al 2017).

Problem solving

It may be necessary to intervene to speed up the birth if there is:
+   concern about the fetal heart rate, fetal tone or colour;
+   delay of more than 5 minutes from emergence of the buttocks; or
+   delay of more than 3 minutes from the emergence of the umbilicus.
Delay is likely to be due to extended arms or neck.

Episiotomy

This surgical intervention should be performed only in 'selected' cases (Impey et al 2017) to create room for emergency procedures if the baby cannot be born spontaneously. An episiotomy should be performed only after discussion with the woman and subsequent verbal consent. If possible, such a discussion should take place before the second stage of labour and not during a contraction. If the woman does not have an epidural in place, the perineum should be infiltrated with local anaesthetic and given time to take effect. It would be very difficult and dangerous to attempt an episiotomy after emergence of the body.

Delay of the fetal head

The Mauriceau–Smelllie–Veit (MSV) manoeuvre is useful when there is delay in the descent of the head, with the purpose of aiding flexion and controlled delivery of the head. An extended head is suspected when the body has emerged and suspended but the nape of the neck does not emerge.

Fig. 4.6A shows how, with the mother in the semi-recumbent position, the dominant hand is placed under the baby's body with its legs on either side of the midwife's arm. A finger (index and ring fingers) is positioned on each cheekbone. The non-dominant hand is used to flex the fetal head by inserting the middle finger into the vagina on to the occiput while the index and ring fingers are positioned on each shoulder. Downward traction is applied via the shoulders until the nape of the neck emerges. Then the baby is lifted upwards so that the head pivots under the symphysis pubis, taking care to keep the head and body in line. Once the face is free the baby can breathe. The vault of the head should then be born slowly. Fig. 4.6B and C shows how in the all-fours position gentle upward pressure is applied to the occiput to flex the head followed by downward pressure on the cheeks. The Burns–Marshall method is also described in the literature but is no longer advocated for fear of damage to the fetal neck (Impey et al 2017). Forceps are sometimes used when an obstetrician conducts the birth with the aim of protecting the head and controlling the speed at which it emerges.

If the woman consents to an intramuscular injection of an oxytocic drug, this should be administered *after* the baby is born.

Activity

- What are the risks to the baby of rapid expulsion of the head?
- What is the Bracht manouvre and when is it used?

Release of the legs

Sometimes the legs are slow to be released, and gentle pressure behind the baby's knees can help flex the knee to aid delivery of the leg, which should be swept across the abdomen. This should be done only if there is delayed progress and a reason to expedite the birth.

Extended arms

If the elbows are not on the chest after the emergence of the umbilicus, one or both arms are extended and can be birthed using the Lövset manoeuvre. With the woman in a semi-recumbent position, the midwife's thumbs are placed on the fetal sacrum and the fingers around the iliac

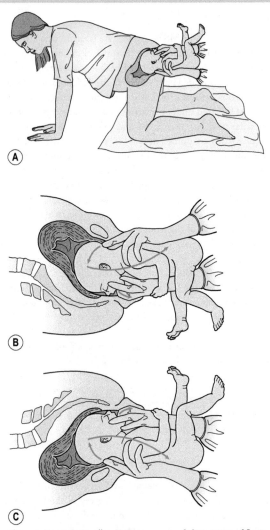

Fig. 4.6 Maurice–Smellie–Veit manoeuvre. **(A)** Direction of flexion in recumbent position and **(B, C)** Direction of flexion in all-fours position. (With permission from Marshall J, Raynor M, eds., Myles Textbook for Midwives, 16th ed., p. 383, Fig. 17.10. Edinburgh: Churchill Livingstone/Elsevier.)

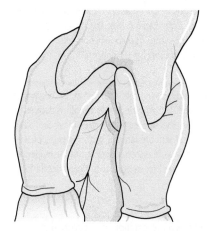

Fig. 4.7 Grasp for Lovset manoeuvre. (With permission from Marshall J, Raynor M, eds., Myles Textbook for Midwives, 16th ed., p. 384, Fig. 17.12. Edinburgh: Churchill Livingstone/Elsevier.)

Table 4.2: **Maternal, fetal and midwifery positions**

Maternal position	Fetal position	Midwife position
All-fours, kneeling	Abdomen uppermost	Behind the woman
Semi-recumbent, sitting	Back uppermost	In front of the woman

crests (see Fig. 4.7). Care must be taken not to grasp the baby around the abdomen, as this could cause damage to the liver or spleen. Downward traction is applied until the axilla can be seen. The baby is turned so that the back is uppermost (see Table 4.2) and through 180 degrees to the opposite side. The anterior arm can now be delivered by flexing the elbow and sweeping the arm across the chest. Rotating the baby back to the other side, keeping the back uppermost, will enable the other arm to enter the pelvis and be birthed in the same way as the first.

REFLECTION ON THE TRIGGER SCENARIO

Look back on the trigger scenario at the start of the chapter.

The ambulance man pushed Julie through the labour ward doors in a wheelchair. She was 37 weeks pregnant with her second baby and in

> established labour. 'I want to push!' she shouted. The midwife showed
> them into a labour room and helped Julie out of the chair. She leaned
> over the bed, pushing involuntarily. After that contraction Julie said, 'The
> last time I saw my midwife she thought he was breech.'

This scenario is one that could face any midwife, just at the beginning
of a shift, with little warning. It highlights the needs for all midwives to
be confident and competent in the safe care of women whose baby
presents by the breech. Now that you are familiar with the principles of
care you should have insight into how the scenario relates to the evidence.
The jigsaw model will now be used to explore the trigger scenario in
more depth.

Effective communication

Caring for a woman with a breech presentation in the second stage of
labour requires precise and effective communication with the maternity
care team and with the woman and her partner. Senior members of the
midwifery and obstetric team would need to be informed immediately
that a breech presentation was confirmed and concurrent record keeping
started and maintained.

Questions that arise from the scenario might include: Had the
woman already telephoned the maternity unit to inform them she was
in labour? Had she communicated her potential breech presentation? Was
it documented in the handheld record that the presentation was possibly
breech? What action plan had the community midwife initiated? What
information had the woman and her partner already been given about
breech birth?

Woman-centred care

What happens next in relation to Julie's care should be the result of joint
decision making. Although the course of action that may need to be
taken will need to be determined rapidly in these circumstances, Julie
should still be central to and involved in the appraisal of the options
available.

Questions that arise from the scenario might include: What information
will the midwife need to glean from Julie that might contribute to the
management of her care? How will Julie's previous birth experience
influence her expectations for this birth? What options will be available
to Julie for pain relief? Does Julie have a birth plan? What efforts can be
made to ensure that she is able to follow through on her hopes and
aspirations for this birth?

Using best evidence

New knowledge is constantly being gained regarding the safest way to care for a woman whose baby presents by the breech. Such knowledge becomes enshrined in national professional guidance and filters down into locally adopted pathways. However, there is often a delay from the publication of the results of groundbreaking research to it becoming accepted as 'this is the way we do things here'.

Questions that arise from the scenario might include: Is there an evidence-based pathway to support care of women who are in the second stage of labour with a fetus presenting by the breech? If so, how has it been communicated to staff? What outmoded practices have been discarded in the light of new knowledge? Are all professionals sufficiently skilled to implement the guidance? What is the evidence regarding the optimum maternal position for breech birth? What is the evidence to support the use of continuous fetal monitoring in these circumstances?

Professional and legal issues

Professional guidance requires the midwife to 'maintain the knowledge and skills you need for safe and effective practice' (NMC 2015: 7). It is her duty to attend breech birth training and the employer's responsibility to provide it. Midwives also need to be aware of their responsibility with regard to seeking informed consent before any procedures or interventions. Having ensured that a woman understands the implications of the choices available, she must also respect a woman's right to decline treatments.

Questions that arise from the scenario might include: When did the midwife last attend for her emergency skills and drills update? Did it include hands-on preparation for management of a breech baby with extended arms with a woman in the all-fours position? What other methods can the midwife use to ensure she keeps up to date with assisted breech birth? What are the implications of performing an episiotomy without consent? If Julie declined fetal monitoring, how would the midwife respond and what actions would she take?

Team working

The team of professionals who care for women in labour extends outside the bounds of the maternity unit. Ensuring that they all work together effectively requires effective communication and continuous learning from individual case studies and national confidential enquires.

Questions that arise from the scenario might include: Did ambulance control phone through to labour ward that they were bringing in a woman in labour with a suspected breech presentation? What opportunities are there for shared learning between emergency services and maternity units? What are the barriers to effective teamwork across disciplines? Who is the lead professional for a woman with a breech presentation? Is there the facility for Julie to have an ultrasound scan in labour, and when might this be advisable? How many other professionals might be involved in Julie's care? What opportunities are there for team debriefing after the birth?

Clinical dexterity

The midwife needs to use very specific midwifery skills in this scenario. She needs to be able to undertake an accurate vaginal examination and confirm presentation, position, descent and cervical dilatation. She needs to have a working knowledge of the female anatomy in order to provide continuous care to Julie irrespective of which position she adopts for pushing and for birth. The midwife needs to be able to recognize if the fetus becomes compromised and take the appropriate action.

Questions that arise from the scenario might include: What opportunities are there for developing and maintaining clinical skills outside of annual skills and drills updates? How can student midwives acquire and practise their clinical labour ward skills? What is the role of the student midwife's mentor in relation to her skill acquisition? What systems are in place where you work for recently qualified midwives to receive senior support and supervision?

Models of care

With the publication of the Peel Report (Department of Health 1970) came the recommendation that all births should take place in hospital. Before that, birth in community settings had been steadily declining and at the same time birth outcomes were improving. It was therefore assumed that birth in hospital was the safest option. Since then, there has been a range of maternity policy documents (Department of Health 1993, 2004, 2007; National Maternity Review 2016) advocating that women should have a choice with regard to the place where they give birth. However, this choice must be informed by current evidence, the woman must be aware of the risk and benefits of the various models available. When a woman is having midwifery-led care and a breech presentation is confirmed, the obstetric team should be informed.

Questions that arise from the scenario might include: Why did Julie choose to have her second baby in a maternity unit? What did Birth Place Study conclude about the impact of place of birth on maternal and neonatal outcomes? Is there a specialist breech team in the maternity unit where you work? When a woman is having midwifery-led care and a breech presentation is confirmed, how is care transferred to the consultant unit where you work? Does the community midwife continue to provide care?

Safe environment

The RCOG Green-top Guideline (Impey et al 2017) recommends that women who are having a baby who presents by the breech should be cared for in a hospital 'with facilities for immediate caesarean section'. It does not recommend that birth should routinely be facilitated in a theatre environment.

Questions that arise from the scenario might include: What precautionary measures can be put in place to ensure that Julie and her baby receive prompt and effective care if the baby's condition becomes compromised during labour or birth? How many minutes does it take to transfer a woman to the theatre from your labour ward? What systems are there to support the midwife to feel safe in her practice when caring for a woman with a breech presentation? How can the woman's psychological safety needs be met? What environmental factors will promote the likelihood of a physiological birth?

Promotes health

The birth of a baby is a life-changing event irrespective of its presentation as it emerges into the world. Although it will be prudent to involve senior midwifery and medical colleagues in the preparations for a breech birth, it is important to remember that the parents should be central to the event. They will be meeting their new baby for the first time, and all efforts should be made to promote a calm and respectful environment that is conducive to loving parent–infant interaction.

Questions that arise from the scenario might include: How can the environment be adapted to help Julie feel calm while ensuring that safety is maintained? What additional observations might be required to be made on babies born by the breech? How can Julie be prepared for how her baby might behave in the first 24 hours? Who should perform the first examination of the newborn screening? Will any follow-up investigations need to be offered for Julie's baby?

Further scenarios

The following scenarios enable you to consider how specific situations influence the care the midwife provides. Use the jigsaw model to explore the issues raised in the scenario.

SCENARIO 1

Amina is expecting her first baby and has now reached 32 weeks' gestation. She has been having some irregular contractions, which are now becoming more painful and closer together. She rings the local maternity unit and is advised to attend to be checked out. She is seen by Lou, the registrar, and premature labour is confirmed, as Amina's cervix is 6 centimetres dilated. Lou is unsure of the presentation, as Amina is unable to tolerate further examination; however, ultrasound confirms the baby is coming bottom first.

Practice point

We know that perinatal morbidity and mortality are higher in babies who are born prematurely whether they are presenting by the breech or not. The evidence suggests that for premature babies presenting by the breech in spontaneous labour, vaginal birth should be considered, depending on the availability of a skilled practitioner. However, if early delivery is being planned because there is concern about the fetus or mother, planned caesarean is the mode of choice for birth (Impey et al 2017).

Questions that arise from the scenario might include: Does Amina have any risk factors associated with a predisposition to preterm birth? Has Amina's pregnancy been uneventful to this point? What ultrasound measurements, other than presentation, are useful to inform the management plan for Amina? What blood tests might the registrar request? What other investigations might be considered to identify the potential cause of premature labour?

SCENARIO 2

Sarah is 37 weeks pregnant and expecting twins. She visits the maternity unit for serial growth scans and her scan showed that the first baby was now presenting by the breech. Her consultant recommends an elective caesarean and would like to book it for the following day. Sarah had hoped for a vaginal birth.

Practice point

About 40% of twin pregnancies will continue to term, and delivery from 37 weeks is recommended (National Institute for Health and Care Excellence 2011). The RCOG Green-top Guidance (Impey et al 2017) recommends that, although the evidence is limited, elective caesarean is recommended when the first twin is presenting by the breech. However, if labour is spontaneous, emergency caesarean should not be routinely offered, unless no operator skilled in vaginal breech birth is available and/or there are other risk factors.

Questions that arise from the scenario might include: How can this evidence be best presented to Sarah? Why is it recommended that she have an elective caesarean? What are the potential risks associated with a breech first twin? What are the risks to Sarah of caesarean birth? If she wishes to continue with her pregnancy and wait events, how should her care be managed?

Conclusion

During a breech birth the midwife needs to remain calm and continue to monitor the well-being of the woman and her baby. She needs to alert the relevant members of the multiprofessional team and work with them to achieve an optimum outcome. Where progress is steady and the fetal condition remains good, she or he should keep her hands off the breech and observe the woman birth her baby. When progress is slow or there is evidence of fetal compromise, she should act competently to assist the woman in her efforts.

Resources

Birth on all fours (photos)

Wildschut, H., van Belzen-Slappendel, H., Jans, S., 2017. The art of vaginal breech birth at term on all fours. Clin. Case Rep. 5, 182–186.

Breech birth photos

Cronk, M., 1998. Hands off the breech. Pract. Midwife 1, 13–15.

Cronk, M., 1998. Midwives and breech births. Pract. Midwife 1, 44–45.

Counselling women with undiagnosed breech in labour

Walker, S., 2013. Undiagnosed breech: towards a woman-centred approach. Br. J. Midwifery 21, 316–322.

Developmental dysplasia of the hips

Shorter, D., Hong, T., Osborn, D.A., 2011. Screening programmes for developmental dysplasia of the hip in newborn infants. Cochrane Database Syst. Rev. (9), CD004595, doi:10.1002/14651858.CD004595.pub2.

External cephalic version

Hutton, E.K., Hofmeyr, G.J., Dowswell, T., 2015. External cephalic version for breech presentation before term. Cochrane Database Syst. Rev. (7), CD000084, doi:10.1002/14651858.CD000084.pub3.

Place of birth in UK over time

Office for National Statistics (ONS). Home births in the UK: 1955 to 2006.

Nove, A., Berrington, A., Matthews, Z., 2008. Home births in the UK, 1955-2006. Popul. Trends 133, 20–27. Available at: www.ons.gov.uk/ons/rel/population -trends-rd/population-trends/no--133--autumn-2008/home-births-in-the-uk --1955-to-2006.pdf.

References

Bogner, G., Strobl, M., Schausberger, C., et al., 2015. Breech delivery in the all fours position: a prospective observational comparative study with classic assistance. J. Perinat. Med. 43, 707–713.

Department of Health, 1970. The Peel Report. Her Majesty's Stationary Service, London.

Department of Health, 1993. Changing Childbirth: Report of the Expert Maternity Group. Her Majesty's Stationary Service, London.

Department of Health, 2004. National Service Framework for Children, Young People and Maternity Services. Her Majesty's Stationary Office, London.

Department of Health, 2007. Maternity Matters: Choice, Access and Continuity of Care in a Safe Service. Her Majesty's Stationary Office, London.

Downe, S., Marshall, J., 2014. Physiology and care during transition and second stage phases of labour. In: Marshall, J., Raynor, M. (Eds.), Myles Textbook for Midwives, sixteenth ed. Churchill Livingstone/ Elsevier, Edinburgh.

Evans, J., 2012. Understanding physiological breech birth. Essentially MIDIRS. 3, 17–21.

Fahy, K., 2011. Do the findings of the Term Breech Trial apply to spontaneous breech birth? Women Birth 24, 1–2.

Ferreira, J., Borowski, D., Czuba, B., et al., 2015. The evolution of fetal presentation during pregnancy: a retrospective, descriptive cross-sectional study. Acta Obstet. Gynecol. Scand. 94, 660–663.

Goffinet, F., Carayol, M., Foidart, J., et al., PREMODA Study Group, 2006. Is planned vaginal delivery for breech presentation at term still an option? Results of an observational prospective survey in France and Belgium. Am. J. Obstet. Gynecol. 194, 1002–1011.

Hannah, M.E., Hannah, W.J., Hewison, S.A., et al., 2000. Planned caesarean section versus planned vaginal birth for breech presentation at term: a randomised muticentre trial. Lancet 356, 1375–1383.

Impey, L., Murphy, D., Griffiths, M., Penna, L.K., on behalf of the Royal College of Obstetricians and Gynaecologists, 2017. Management of breech presentation. (Green-top guideline No. 20b). BJOG 124, e151–e177. Available at: https:// www.rcog.org.uk/en/guidelines-research-services/guidelines/gtg20b/.

National Institute for Health and Care Excellence (NICE). 2014. updated 2016. Intrapartum care for healthy women and babies. NICE CG190. https:// www.nice.org.uk/guidance/cg190.

National Maternity Review. 2016. Better Births. Improving outcomes of maternity services in England. Available at: https://www.england.nhs.uk/wp-content/ uploads/2016/02/national-maternity-review-report.pdf.

Nursing and Midwifery Council, 2015. The code: professional standards of practice and behaviour for nurses and midwives. https://www.nmc.org.uk/globalassets/ sitedocuments/nmc-publications/nmc-code.pdf.

Ressl, B., O'Beirne, M., 2015. Detecting breech presentation before labour: lessons from a low-risk maternity clinic. J. Obstet. Gynaecol. Can. 37, 702–706.

CHAPTER 5

Shoulder dystocia

TRIGGER SCENARIO

'Well done, just breathe, the head is out now', the midwife said reassuringly. 'He looks a good size', she continued, as she eased the perineum over the baby's chin. Caroline let her head flop back on the pillow. She felt as though she had been pushing for hours. She began to feel her next contraction and wearily raised her head and began to push. 'Come on, Caroline, push really hard', the midwife urged. 'I am', she said, 'I am'.

Introduction

Shoulder dystocia is a frightening experience for both the woman and the midwife. It is usually unexpected, with more than 50% of cases occurring in babies of normal birth weight (Gobbo & Baxley 2000). The midwife needs to know how to deal with this emergency to reduce the likelihood of maternal and neonatal morbidity. This chapter describes the steps the midwife can take to manage shoulder dystocia.

Definition

Many definitions have been put forward to describe shoulder dystocia ranging from those that suggest a time frame for birth of the shoulders after emergence of the head, to those implying 'difficulty' and 'tight fit' (Hansen & Chauhan 2014). Although a universal definition has not been adopted, The Royal College of Obstetricians and Gynaecologists (RCOG) Green-top Guideline (2012, reviewed 2017) offers a more precise description of shoulder dystocia:

> 'vaginal cephalic delivery that requires additional obstetric manoeuvres to deliver the fetus after the head has delivered and gentle traction has failed' (RCOG 2012: 2).

Incidence and risk factors

Shoulder dystocia is a rare occurrence estimated to occur in 0.15% to 2% of vaginal births (Hill & Cohen 2016); however, the incidence increases with fetal weight. In a retrospective analysis of 175,886 births in California

Box 5.1 **Risk factors for shoulder dystocia**

Maternal risk factors	Intrapartum 'alert' factors
Previous obstetric history of shoulder dystocia	Slow progress during labour
Diabetes/gestational diabetes	Need for instrumental delivery
Obesity/excessive weight gain during pregnancy	Fetal chin does not clear the perineum / 'turtle' sign

(Nesbitt et al 1999), it was reported that the incidence of shoulder dystocia in spontaneous births to nondiabetic women was 3% for babies weighing more than 3500 grams; 5.2% for babies weighing 4000 to 4250 grams; and 21.1% for babies weighing 4750 to 5000 grams.

Several factors have been associated with shoulder dystocia, including high maternal weight gain during pregnancy, multiparity and a previous large baby (Geary et al 1995). In the study of Nesbitt et al (1999), women with diabetes had increased odds of 1.7 for shoulder dystocia, while women who had an assisted birth had increased odds of 1.9.

In a retrospective case control study (Larson and Mandelbaum 2013) asymmetrical macrosomia (large body size compared with head circumference) was associated with an increased incidence of shoulder dystocia. Poorly controlled maternal diabetes will predispose the fetus to macrosomia, and the potential for disproportionate distribution of fetal adipose tissue, which places these babies at higher risk than those of equal weight (Hill & Cohen 2016).

In a study involving 8010 first births (Mehta et al 2004), 22% of the women who had shoulder dystocia had a second stage of labour that lasted more than 2 hours compared with 3% of women who did not have shoulder dystocia. Delayed progress in labour should therefore alert the midwife that there is an increased likelihood of shoulder dystocia after the delivery of the head. However, the majority of cases of shoulder dystocia occur when there are no major risk factors (see Box 5.1) (Mehta & Sokol 2014).

Prevention of shoulder dystocia

The only sure way to prevent shoulder dystocia and associated maternal neonatal morbidity is caesarean birth (Mehta & Sokol 2014). Although there are known risk factors, shoulder dystocia is notoriously difficult to predict (Palatnik et al 2016); therefore such a drastic course of action could not be warranted without a specific justification.

Estimating fetal weight by ultrasound scanning at term is one potential way of identifying pregnancies at risk of culminating in shoulder dystocia. Labour could then be induced in high-risk pregnancies. However, antenatal estimation of fetal weight is often imprecise and could lead to unnecessary intervention. In a systematic review of the evidence (Boulvain et al 2016), it was concluded that although induction of labour for suspected macrosomia does result in a lower mean birth weight, a reduced incidence of shoulder dystocia and fewer fractures, it needs to be balanced against increased perineal trauma and neonatal jaundice. Further research is needed to clarify if the benefits of early induction of labour are of clinical benefit.

A randomized controlled trial was conducted (Beall et al 2003) to explore the prophylactic use of the McRobert's manoeuvre (see HELPERR mnemonic later) and suprapubic pressure in women whose babies were estimated to weigh 3800 grams or more. There was no difference between the prophylactic and control groups for head to body birth times, birth injuries or rates of admission to a special care baby unit.

In 2005 an American study was conducted to explore the cost-effectiveness of three techniques for managing fetal macrosomia with a view to reducing the incidence of shoulder dystocia and subsequent brachial plexus injuries (Herbst 2005). Using decision analysis techniques and comparing the cost of three options (elective caesarean, induction of labour or expectant management), it was concluded that expectant management was the most cost-effective approach to care.

Activity

Conduct an Internet search for 'birth after shoulder dystocia'. Look at what mothers are asking each other and how they feel about their experiences.

Management of shoulder dystocia

The management of shoulder dystocia must be prompt and with the ultimate aim of dislodging the fetal shoulder from behind the maternal symphysis pubis, as summed up by Stitely and Gherman (2014) in Box 5.2. This can be achieved by:

External manoeuvres

+ **The McRobert's manoeuvre:** Increasing the anterio-posterior diameter of the maternal pelvis
+ **Suprapubic pressure:** Reducing the fetal bisacromial diameter

Internal manoeuvres

+ **Removal of the posterior arm:** Reducing the diameter of the fetal shoulders by the width of arm
+ **Rotation of the fetal shoulder:** Dislodging the shoulder from behind the symphysis pubis

Box 5.2 **Summary of shoulder dystocia management**

> *The overall goal of shoulder dystocia management is to convert the fetal shoulders to an oblique diameter in order to relieve the obstruction before the fetal brain suffers irreversible hypoxic–ischemic injury.*

(Stitely & Gherman 2014: 194)

Box 5.3 **The HELPERR mnemonic**

H Help – call for appropriate help immediately
E Episiotomy – evaluate for episiotomy
L Legs – assist woman to put legs in the McRobert's position
P Pressure – apply lateral supra pubic pressure to fetal shoulders
E Enter – enter the vagina and undertake internal manoeuvres
R Remove – remove posterior arm
R Roll – roll on to hands and knees

The mnemonic debate

There are many algorithms (e.g. RCOG 2012) and mnemonics (e.g. Draycott et al 2008) available in the literature and incorporated into trust guidelines that are designed to support healthcare professionals in clinical practice. Many trusts use the protocol described and taught on the Advanced Life Support in Obstetrics (ALSO) course for the management of shoulder dystocia (Gobbo & Baxley 2000). It is therefore appropriate that student midwives become familiar with this drill.

Although the mnemonic HELPERR is part of the protocol, the sequence of events may change depending on the individual circumstances (Hill & Cohen 2016). For example, if the woman is agile and able to easily turn over to an all-fours position, this may facilitate delivery of the posterior shoulder without the need to use internal manoeuvres. However, it may be the case, especially in a labour that has been protracted, that the woman may have an epidural in situ and be relatively immobile.

The HELPERR mnemonic (Box 5.3) is useful to help some practitioners remember a list of useful techniques in a logical order and is therefore used as a familiar framework for presentation of the emergency techniques in this chapter. However, it is should be seen as a 'menu of options' (Samples 2018) rather than a prescriptive sequence of events. The most important aspect of learning how to manage shoulder dystocia is knowing what to try first and how to perform that skill. Learning the precise name of a technique or reciting a mnemonic should not be the priority (RCOG 2012). The names of the different techniques are presented in the following description, for the student's information, as she will encounter these throughout her education programme. Regular practice of the techniques involved should be facilitated with the multi-professional team using mannequins, and targeted training has been shown to improve outcomes (Allen et al 2017).

H – Help

As soon as shoulder dystocia is diagnosed, maternal pushing should be discouraged and the midwife must summon appropriate help in accordance with the Nursing and Midwifery Council (NMC) Code (2015). The method for doing this will vary from unit to unit, as some will have a particular emergency buzzer or other means of alerting staff that an emergency has arisen. Student midwives should familiarize themselves with the means of calling assistance in each placement in which they work, as they may be asked to raise the alarm.

E – Episiotomy, evaluate for

Shoulder dystocia is not caused by soft tissue resistance but by the impaction of the fetal shoulder against the maternal symphysis pubis. As such, an episiotomy will not resolve shoulder dystocia but it can make it easier to undertake manipulative internal manoeuvres. Taking a few seconds to *consider* the possibility of performing an episiotomy if internal procedures were to be required is what should be evaluated at this point. An episiotomy should not be undertaken unless internal manoeuvres are required (RCOG 2012). Performing an episiotomy after the birth of the head is not an easy procedure, and there is no consensus regarding the wisdom of making one to expedite the birth. Indeed, a study of 953 shoulder dystocias over a 10-year period showed that the rate of brachial plexus injuries did not change over time despite a reduction in the episiotomy rate with shoulder dystocia from 40% to 4% (Paris et al 2011).

L – Legs: McRobert's manoeuvre

If the woman has her legs in lithotomy position, she should be assisted to bring both legs out of the supports simultaneously by a helper on either side. Any pillows should be removed, the woman should be assisted to lie flat and both legs taken to knee-to-abdomen position through flexion and abduction of her hips (see Fig. 5.1).

This simple procedure is associated with the relief of 42% of cases of shoulder dystocia, and is therefore recommended as the first line of action to be taken (Gherman et al 1997). As a simulated squatting position (the woman's thighs flexed against her abdomen), the anterior–posterior diameters of the pelvis are increased, allowing it to rotate over the fetal shoulder. After adoption of this position, a further attempt to birth the baby should be made, using normal traction in line with the fetal spine.

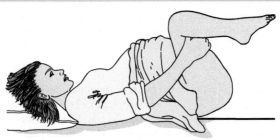

Fig. 5.1 The position for the McRobert's manoeuvre. (With permission from Marshall J, Raynor M, eds., Myles Textbook for Midwives, 16th ed., p. 480, Fig. 22.5. Edinburgh: Churchill Livingstone/Elsevier.)

P – Pressure: suprapubic

In an attempt to dislodge the impacted shoulder from the symphysis pubis, an assistant should locate the fetal back and apply lateral pressure to the posterior aspect of the fetal shoulder. The application of pressure is also known as the Rubin's I manoeuvre and is best achieved using the heel of one hand over the other, as when performing cardiac massage (Gobbo & Baxley 2000). At first the pressure should be constant while the midwife continues gentle traction, but if this is not successful a gentle rocking motion can be tried. Again, a further attempt to birth the baby should be made, using normal traction in line with the fetal spine, to see if this has worked.

E – Enter: internal manoeuvres

Three manoeuvres can be attempted to rotate the anterior shoulder into an oblique plane and then under the maternal symphysis. The sacral hollow is where the pelvis is most spacious and the whole hand should be inserted; this is often described as the Pringle hand (Draycott et al 2008):

1. **The Rubin's II manoeuvre** (Fig. 5.2) This process will adduct the fetal shoulders. The fingers are inserted into the vagina and pressure applied behind the anterior shoulder towards the fetal chest. If the shoulders are successfully rotated into the oblique plane, birth should be re-attempted. If not, try the second manoeuvre.

2. **The wood screw manoeuvre** This process abducts the posterior fetal shoulder. While maintaining the position for Rubin's (II), the midwife inserts her second hand into the vagina and locates the anterior aspect of the posterior shoulder. Pressure is then applied in the same direction as for Rubin's (II). If the shoulders are successfully rotated into the oblique plane, delivery should be re-attempted. If not, try the third manoeuvre.

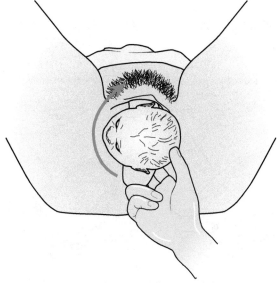

Fig. 5.2 The Rubin's manoeuvre. (With permission from Marshall J, Raynor M, eds., Myles Textbook for Midwives, 16th ed., p. 481, Fig. 22.7. Edinburgh: Churchill Livingstone/Elsevier.)

3. **Reverse wood screw** This process rotates the baby in the opposite direction. The midwife will need to change hands; this time fingers are placed behind the posterior shoulder and pressure is applied to turn the baby 180 degrees in the opposite direction. Delivery of the baby is then re-attempted.

R – Remove (deliver) the posterior arm

This internal manoeuvre is increasingly being advocated as an earlier option (Poggi et al 2003). By delivering the posterior arm (Fig. 5.3), the anterior shoulder can drop into the pelvis. The midwife needs to insert her hand into the vagina to locate the posterior fetal arm. The elbow should then be located and flexed to draw it across the chest wall. The hand should be delivered first. The fetus often rotates as the arm is delivered, freeing the shoulder and enabling the baby to be born.

R – Roll the woman on to all-fours

Also known as the 'Gaskin' manoeuvre, helping a woman to adopt an 'all-fours' position has been shown to be an effective means of resolving

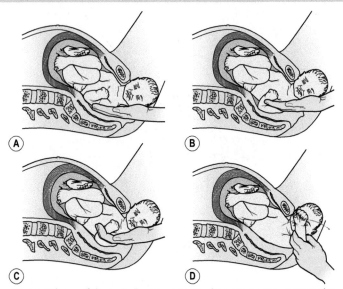

Fig. 5.3 Delivery of the posterior arm. **A** Locate the posterior arm. **B** Direct the arm into the sacral hollow. **C** Grasp the wrist and forearm. **D** Sweep the arm over the chest and deliver the hand. (With permission from Marshall J, Raynor M, eds., Myles Textbook for Midwives, 16th ed., p. 482, Fig. 22.9A–D. Edinburgh: Churchill Livingstone/Elsevier.)

shoulder dystocia, with a minimal incidence of either maternal or neonatal complications (Bruner et al 1998).

Moving the woman into this position may dislodge the fetal shoulder and enable the birth to be facilitated. The woman will need a great deal of support to change position, especially if she has an epidural, catheter, fetal monitoring and/or intravenous infusion. The midwife should then attempt to deliver the posterior shoulder first (which is now nearest the ceiling), using gentle downward traction. The internal manoeuvres can also be tried in this position.

Activity

Read: Ansell L, McAra-Couper J, Smythe E. 2012. Shoulder dystocia: a qualitative exploration of what works. Midwifery 28:e521–e528.

Consider the role of 'axillary traction' as a tool in the management of shoulder dystocia.

'Last resort' manoeuvres

1. **Clavicular fracture** By applying pressure in the middle of the clavicle, the bone will break – thus reducing the breadth of the shoulders.
2. **The Zavanelli manoeuvre** The head is replaced into the vagina by reversing the mechanism of birth. The baby is then born by caesarean.
3. **Muscle relaxation** Either uterine or musculoskeletal muscle relaxation is induced using drug therapy.
4. **Hysterotomy** An abdominal incision is made, hysterotomy performed and the shoulders rotated transabdominally to facilitate vaginal birth.
5. **Symphysiotomy** Division of the cartilage of the symphysis pubis.
    It should be noted that the following approaches should *not* be taken:
*   **Never** apply fundal pressure.
*   **Never** apply excessive traction on the fetal head.
*   **Never** attempt to rotate the fetus by its head.

Activity

*   Find out what drugs can be used to induce uterine or musculoskeletal muscle relaxation.
*   What is meant by the term 'tocolysis'?

Potential complications after shoulder dystocia
Maternal

The mother and her birth partner may be emotionally traumatized after shoulder dystocia. They should be given the opportunity to go through the events when they are rested and have had time to process what happened.

The mother may sustain soft tissue injury to the vaginal tract, particularly if internal manoeuvres have been employed in an attempt to disimpact the fetal shoulders.

Symphyseal separation and temporary femoral neuropathy have been associated with the McRobert's manoeuvre (Gherman et al 1998). The risk of postpartum haemorrhage is also increased (Gobbo & Baxley 2000). It is difficult to ascertain, in the absence of prospective studies, whether obstetric manoeuvres used during shoulder dystocia increase the risk of urinary incontinence, because they are both linked with high birth weight, assisted birth and multiparity (Mazouni et al 2006). Management of shoulder dystocia that includes the use of episiotomy has been associated with a sevenfold increase in the rate of severe perineal trauma without improving neonatal outcomes (Gurewitsch et al 2004).

Neonatal

The most serious potential complication of shoulder dystocia is hypoxia, leading to death or permanent brain damage.

After delivery of the head, the umbilical cord is compressed between the woman's pelvis and the body of the fetus. There are approximately 7 minutes to facilitate the birth before a previously noncompromised baby becomes compromised (Gobbo & Baxley 2000).

Activity

- Consider the implications of clamping and cutting a nuchal cord before the shoulders are delivered.
- Find out if symphysiotomy has ever been performed where you work. If so, establish why and what the outcome was.

The most common injuries after shoulder dystocia involve brachial plexus damage, resulting in one of three palsies:

- **Erb's palsy** Results from damage to the fifth and sixth cervical nerve roots. It is often referred to as the 'waiter's tip position' because the elbow is extended, the arm is rotated outwards, the wrist flexed and fingers partially closed, as if the patient were awaiting a discreet payment.
- **Klumpke's palsy** Results from damage to the seventh and eighth cervical and first thoracic nerve roots. This palsy affects the lower half of the arm, giving rise to a limp wrist and paralysed hand.
- **Total brachial plexus palsy** Results from damage to the fifth, sixth, seventh and eighth cervical and first thoracic nerve roots (i.e. the whole brachial plexus). This palsy involves paralysis of the whole arm, with circulatory problems and lack of sensation (Greig 2003).

Occasionally, the baby sustains a fracture of the clavicle or humerus during the birth after shoulder dystocia. Both of these fractures usually heal without any long-term problems.

Activity

- How does brachial plexus injury develop?
- What is the incidence of brachial plexus injury to the neonate after a case of shoulder dystocia?
- What proportion of brachial plexus injuries are permanent?

Documentation

The importance of detailed documentation of action taken after the diagnosis of shoulder dystocia cannot be over-emphasized. One member of the team should be assigned to note down key times, including when help was summoned, when and who came and when each procedure was attempted. It can take many years for a claim to come to court, after which time the midwife may have only a vague memory of what happened when and who was called for assistance. It is recommended that a structured proforma be used (Crofts et al 2008) to facilitate this, and these should be available in all birth settings. It is usual practice to complete an incident form after shoulder dystocia so that the circumstances of the case can be looked at in detail by the maternity governance and clinical leads.

Carr (2004) describes two cases in which babies suffered Erb's palsy following shoulder dystocia. In the first case, excellent record-keeping provided sufficient evidence that the midwife had taken appropriate action and the case was successfully defended. In the second case, however, the practitioners involved in the ventouse birth could not remember the details surrounding the incident. The documentation did not provide sufficient evidence of appropriate care, and the court found in favour of the claimant.

Activity

Access the RCOG (2012) guidelines on shoulder dystocia. Look at the proforma for documentation and consider how it compares to the documentation where you work.

REFLECTION ON THE TRIGGER SCENARIO

Look back on the trigger scenario at the start of the chapter.

'Well done, just breathe, the head is out now', the midwife said reassuringly. 'He looks a good size', she continued, as she eased the perineum over the baby's chin. Caroline let her head flop back on the pillow. She felt as though she had been pushing for hours. She began to feel her next contraction and wearily raised her head and began to push. 'Come on, Caroline, push really hard', the midwife urged. 'I am', she said, 'I am'.

This scenario, in which the baby's head is delivered but there is delay in delivery of the shoulders, is one that any student of midwife could face without warning. Now that you are familiar with the management of shoulder dystocia you will have insight into how the scenario relates to evidence for best practice in this situation. The jigsaw model will now be used to explore the trigger scenario in more depth.

Effective communication

It is important that the midwife continues to communicate effectively with the woman, her birth partner and maternity care team in order to achieve a successful resolution to shoulder dystocia. This is a high-adrenaline situation where every second counts to ensure that the baby is born without neurological damage.

Questions that arise from the scenario might include: What should the midwife say to the woman? How can the birth partner help in this situation? Who else must the midwife communicate with and how? When help arrives, what key information should the midwife report to them? When and how should the sequence of events be documented?

Woman-centred care

Ensuring that the woman and her birth partner remain central, the management of shoulder dystocia is important not only from a social and emotional point of view, but also to enable them to engage with the necessary steps to resolve the situation. The woman should be involved in the process and asked to listen carefully for instructions. She should be advised not to push and helped to do this by her partner. If she is mobile and was previously in a semirecumbent position, she can be helped into an all-fours position to facilitate delivery of the posterior shoulder. Keeping her focused and engaged in the process will help all involved to remain calm and working as a team to best effect.

Questions that arise from the scenario might include: Caroline is tired after a long second stage of labour; how can the midwife motivate her to assist with the management of this emergency situation? After the birth, how should Caroline be debriefed about what happened? How will her community midwife be informed about this complication of second stage in order to continue the emotional support Caroline may need?

Using best evidence

New knowledge is constantly emerging about the most effective ways to provide emergency maternity care. It is a professional requirement to keep up to date with changes in practice and to ensure that we provide evidence-based care where this is information is available (NMC 2015).

Questions that arise from the scenario might include: What national professional guidance supports our practice when caring for a woman with shoulder dystocia? Do local guidelines reflect this evidence base? When were your local guidelines about the management of shoulder dystocia last updated? Who was involved in that process, and do they reflect contemporary knowledge?

Professional and legal issues

The effective management of shoulder dystocia is scrutinized, following the routine reporting of the event to the maternity unit's governance lead. This is to ensure that the correct processes were followed, especially in the event of significant consequences for the woman or her baby. It may be necessary for the midwife involved to review her documentation and ensure that all actions were documented in line with NMC standards. Reviewing the care in this way enables the team to learn from this reflection and for additional education or training to be facilitated.

Questions that arise from the scenario might include: How are incidents reported where you work? Who looks at incident notifications, and what process is then followed? How many incidences of shoulder dystocia are reported each year where you work?

Team working

Once the midwife suspects shoulder dystocia, she should call for help using the appropriate system that will request immediate response from a team that includes an obstetrician, senior midwifery colleagues and a paediatrician. In units where multi-professional training is in place, colleagues will be used to working with each other and taking on appropriate roles that have been practised in scenarios with the use of manikins. However, every midwife must be prepared to undertake all procedures necessary, just in case an obstetrician is unavailable at that crucial time.

Questions that arise from the scenario might include: In what situations might the midwife need to perform internal manoeuvres? Who should the midwife call if she is faced with a shoulder dystocia during a home birth? How can maternity support workers provide support when shoulder dystocia occurs in the maternity unit? Which member of the multi-professional team is responsible for checking the resuscitaire is fully stocked in working order where you work?

Clinical dexterity

The ability to provide safe and effective care to a woman who is experiencing shoulder dystocia depends on the midwife's ability to implement a range of clinical skills. She needs to have a working knowledge of the woman's anatomy and be able to adapt her care depending on the position of the woman and the clinical circumstances she finds herself in.

Questions that arise from the scenario might include: If the woman is in a semirecumbent position, how can the midwife help the woman into the McRobert's position? Where should the midwife place her hands when she is asked to perform suprapubic pressure to attempt to adduct the fetal shoulders? Where should she insert her hand in order to initiate internal rotations manoeuvres? What position should the woman be in if an attempt to deliver the posterior shoulder first is being considered?

Models of care

Women who are experiencing a normal pregnancy are usually cared for under midwifery-led care. Most women who experience shoulder dystocia may have had a previously uncomplicated maternity journey. It is maternity care policy (National Maternity Review 2016) that women should be involved in decisions about their care, and this includes place of birth.

Questions that arise from the scenario might include: Was Caroline offered a choice regarding place of birth? If so, what issues did Caroline discuss with her midwife in relation to this important decision? What evidence did the midwife draw on to inform the debate? When is it most appropriate to have these discussions? What antenatal factors might influence who is the lead professional for Caroline?

Safe environment

Caroline has had a long labour and is very tired. She will need much emotional support and expert clinical monitoring to ensure she has the stamina to keep going. Midwives are also at risk of becoming overly tired or dehydrated when caring for women over a long period of time, and such situations have the potential to compromise safety and must therefore be carefully managed.

Questions that arise from the scenario might include: What does the midwife do to ensure that Caroline remains well hydrated and has sufficient energy throughout labour? How is the midwife's health and well-being taken care of during her shift? Has she been the only midwife caring for Caroline? What systems are there to ensure that midwives get adequate rest both during and in between shifts? What facilities are there for birth partners to eat and drink where you work?

Promotes health

Shoulder dystocia can have long-term sequelae for both the woman and her baby. Although the potential for these can be minimized by the implementation of robust evidence-based protocols, the possibility of enduring emotional and physical symptoms cannot be ruled out.

Questions that arise from the scenario might include: How does gestational weight gain affect maternal health? How can the incidence of perineal trauma be reduced during the management of shoulder dystocia? How can the midwife help reduce the risk of the woman developing post-traumatic stress symptoms as a consequence of her birth experience? What services are there for women to discuss the events around their birth, to help them understand and make sense of them?

Further scenarios

The following scenarios enable you to consider how specific situations influence the care the midwife provides. Use the jigsaw model to explore the issues raised in the scenario.

SCENARIO 1

After 5 minutes of manoeuvres to assist the birth of Caroline's baby, her daughter Ava is born pale and floppy. Ava's heart rate is 60 beats per minute, and she is not making any respiratory effort. She is taken by the paediatrician and resuscitated via bag and mask. After administration of inflation breaths, the heart rate increased and she began to cry. However, it is noted that she is not moving her left arm.

Practice point

There is limited time between delivery of the head and the subsequent birth of the baby until the baby may become compromised due to lack of oxygen to the brain. Hence it is important that the management of shoulder dystocia is managed appropriately and without delay. In some cases, the baby may sustain a fracture or palsy as a result of the position it has been in during the labour or the manoeuvres required to expedite the birth.

Questions that arise from the scenario might include:

+   In how many minutes after delivery of the head must the body be born to avoid neurological damage to the baby?
+   How many inflation breaths should be given to a baby who has not made any respiratory effort?
+   What is a normal heart rate for a neonate?
+   What nerves might be damaged in the baby's neck?
+   Is Erb's palsy a permanent condition?
+   What fractures might Ava have sustained?
+   What is the treatment and follow-up for these fractures?

Midwife Lucy has just met Caroline, whose daughter is now five years old, and is about to start her booking history. Caroline sits down and before Lucy can introduce herself she says, 'I want a caesarean this time. I can't go through that again'.

Practice point

Some women who have had a traumatic birth experience will delay becoming pregnant again or even choose to limit their family size to avoid a repeat scenario. Women who have shoulder dystocia in one birth are more likely to experience it again in a subsequent birth (Gurewitsch et al 2007). It is therefore understandable that Caroline has concerns about giving birth again.

Questions that arise from the scenario might include:

+ Had Lucy looked at Caroline's previous obstetric history before she met Caroline for her booking history?
+ Where would this be documented, and is it available in the community setting?
+ Had Caroline had the opportunity to talk to someone about her birth experience in the postnatal period?
+ What additional support can Lucy offer Caroline in this pregnancy?
+ Is previous shoulder dystocia an indication for caesarean birth in a subsequent pregnancy? Should it be?
+ What maternity care pathway should Caroline be referred to?

Conclusion

Shoulder dystocia is a life-threatening emergency and requires swift and appropriate action from the maternity care team. The midwife needs to be equipped with the appropriate clinical skills at her fingertips, so that there is no delay in initiating an evidence-based protocol. She also needs to have a calm demeanour so that she can communicate with the woman and her partner, maintaining their trust and enabling them to help facilitate the birth.

Resources

Shoulder dystocia in the community

Kallianidis, A.F., Smit, M., Van Roosmalen, J., 2016. Shoulder dystocia in primary care in the Netherlands. Acta. Obstet. Gynaecol. Scand. 95, 203–209.

Erb's palsy information and diagrams

https://www.erbs-palsy.co.uk/index.html

Information for women

Royal College of Obstetricians & Gynaecologists (RCOG), 2013. Information for you. Shoulder dystocia. Available at: https://www.rcog.org.uk/globalassets/documents/patients/patient-information-leaflets/pregnancy/pi-shoulder-dystocia.pdf

Evidence base

Gherman, R., 2002. Shoulder dystocia: an evidence-based evaluation of the obstetrical nightmare. Clin. Obstet. Gynecol. 45, 345–362.

Resuscitation of premature infants

Anup, K., Poeltler, D., Durham, J., et al., 2016. Neonatal resuscitation with an intact cord: a randomized clinical trial. J. Pediatr. 178, 75–80.e3.

Shoulder dystocia training – impact

Crofts, J.F., Lenguerrand, E., Bentham, G.L., et al., 2016. Prevention of brachial plexus injury—12 years of shoulder dystocia training: an interrupted time-series study. BJOG. Available at: https://d1oi.org/10.1111/1471-0528.13302

References

Allen, E., Will, S., Allen, R., Satin, A., 2017. Targeted training effort improves shoulder dystocia management and outcomes. Am. J. Obstet. Gynecol. 216, S517.

Beall, M.H., Spong, C.Y., Ross, M.G., 2003. A randomized controlled trial of prophylactic maneuvers to reduce head-to-body delivery time in patients at risk for shoulder dystocia. Obstet. Gynecol. 102, 31–35.

Boulvain, M., Irion, O., Dowswell, T., Thornton, J.G., 2016. Induction of labour at or near term for suspected fetal macrosomia. Cochrane Database Syst. Rev. (5), CD000938, doi:10.1002/14651858.CD000938.pub2.

Bruner, J.P., Drummond, S., Meenan, A.L., Gaskin, I.M., 1998. The all-fours maneuver for reducing shoulder dystocia during labor. J. Reprod. Med. 43, 439–443.

Carr, N., 2004. Litigation and the midwife: shoulder dystocia. Pract. Midwife 7 (24), 26–27.

Crofts, J., Bartlett, C., Ellis, D., et al., 2008. Documentation of simulated shoulder dystocia: accurate and complete? BJOG 115, 1303–1308.

Crofts, J.F., Lenguerrand, E., Bentham, G.L., et al., 2016. Prevention of brachial plexus injury – 12 years of shoulder dystocia training: an interrupted time-series study. BJOG 123, 111–118.

Draycott, T.J., Crofts, J.F., Ash, J.P., et al., 2008. Improving neonatal outcome through practical shoulder dystocia training. Obstet. Gynecol. 112 (1), 14–20.

Geary, M., McParland, P., Johnson, H., Stronge, J., 1995. Shoulder dystocia – is it predictable? Eur. J. Obstet. Gynecol. Reprod. Biol. 62, 15–18.

Gherman, R.B., 2002. Shoulder dystocia: an evidence-based evaluation of the obstetric nightmare. Clin. Obstet. Gynecol. 45, 345–362.

Gherman, R.B., Goodwin, T.W., Souter, I., et al., 1997. The McRobert's maneuver for the alleviation of shoulder dystocia: how successful is it? Am. J. Obstet. Gynecol. 176, 656–661.

Gherman, R.B., Ouzounian, J.G., Incerpi, M.H., Goodwin, T.W., 1998. Symphyseal separation and transient femoral neuropathy associated with the McRobert's maneuver. Am. J. Obstet. Gynecol. 178, 609–610.

Gobbo, R., Baxley, E.G., 2000. Shoulder dystocia. In: ALSO Advanced Life Support in Obstetrics Provider Course Syllabus. American Academy of Family Physicians, Leawood, KS.

Greig, C., 2003. Trauma during birth: haemorrhage and convulsions. In: Fraser, D.M., Cooper, M.A. (Eds.), Myles Textbook for Midwives. Churchill Livingstone/Elsevier, Edinburgh.

Gurewitsch, E.D., Donithan, M., Stallings, S.P., et al., 2004. Episiotomy versus fetal manipulation in managing severe shoulder dystocia: a comparison of outcomes. Am. J. Obstet. Gynecol. 191, 911–916.

Gurewitsch, E.D., Johnson, T.L., Allen, R.H., 2007. After shoulder dystocia: managing the subsequent pregnancy and delivery. Semin. Perinatol. 31 (3), 185–195.

Hansen, A., Chauhan, S.P., 2014. Shoulder dystocia: definitions and incidence. Semin. Perinatol. 38 (4), 184–188. doi:10.1053/j.semperi.2014.04.002.

Herbst, M.A., 2005. Treatment of suspected fetal macrosomia: a cost-effectiveness analysis. Am. J. Obstet. Gynecol. 193 (Pt 2), 1035–1039.

Hill, M.G., Cohen, W.R., 2016. Shoulder dystocia: prediction and management. Womens Health 12, 251–261.

Larson, A., Mandelbaum, D., 2013. Association of head circumference and shoulder dystocia in macrosomic neonates. Matern. Child Health J. 17, 501–504.

Mazouni, C., Menard, J.P., Porcu, G., et al., 2006. Maternal morbidity associated with obstetrical maneuvers in shoulder dystocia. Eur. J. Obstet. Gynecol. Reprod. Biol. 129 (1), 15–18.

Mehta, S.H., Bujold, E., Blackwell, S.C., et al., 2004. Is abnormal labor associated with shoulder dystocia in nulliparous women? Am. J. Obstet. Gynecol. 190, 1604–1609.

Mehta, S., Sokol, R., 2014. Shoulder dystocia: risk factors, predictability, and preventability. Semin. Perinatol. 38, 189–193.

National Maternity Review, 2016. Better Births. Improving outcomes of maternity services in England. Available at: https://www.england.nhs.uk/wp-content/uploads/2016/02/national-maternity-review-report.pdf.

Nesbitt, T.S., Gilbert, W.M., Herrchen, B., 1999. Shoulder dystocia and associated risk factors with macrosomic infants born in California. Am. J. Obstet. Gynecol. 180, 1047.

Nursing and Midwifery Council, 2015. The code: professional standards of practice and behaviour for nurses and midwives. https://www.nmc.org.uk/globalassets/sitedocuments/nmc-publications/nmc-code.pdf.

Palatnik, A., Grobman, W., Hellendag, M., et al., 2016. Predictors of shoulder dystocia at the time of operative vaginal delivery. Am. J. Obstet. Gynecol. 215, 624.e1–624.e5.

Paris, A., Greenberg, J., Ecker, J., McElrath, T., 2011. Is an episiotomy necessary with a shoulder dystocia? Am. J. Obstet. Gynecol. 205, 217.e1–217.e3.

Poggi, S.H., Spong, C.Y., Allen, R., 2003. Prioritizing posterior arm delivery during severe shoulder dystocia. Obstet. Gynecol. 101 (5, Part 2 Suppl.), 1068–1072.

Royal College of Obstetricians & Gynaecologists (RCOG). Shoulder dystocia (Green-top Guideline No. 42). Available at: https://www.rcog.org.uk/en/guidelines-research-services/guidelines/gtg42/.

Samples, J., 2018. Personal Communication.

Stitely, M., Gherman, R., 2014. Shoulder dystocia: management and documentation. Semin. Perinatol. 38, 194–200.

CHAPTER 6

Postpartum haemorrhage

TRIGGER SCENARIO

Debra is holding her new baby skin-to-skin after birth. She starts to shift uncomfortably in the bed. She turns to Emily, the midwife, and says, 'I feel really wet'.

Introduction

Postpartum haemorrhage (PPH) is a potentially life-threatening emergency that requires swift and appropriate action from the midwife. The incidence of PPH is rising globally, and a recent study suggests it could occur in about one-third of births (Briley et al 2014). Recurrence of PPH in subsequent births is also high (Fullerton et al 2013; Oberg et al 2014). Although there are predisposing factors that increase the risk of PPH, many instances of PPH are unanticipated and therefore a shock to both the woman and the midwife. This chapter explores the midwife's role in the diagnosis, care and treatment of primary and secondary PPH.

Definition

The usual definition of PPH is 'a blood loss of 500 ml or more within 24 hours after birth, while severe or major PPH is defined as a blood loss of 1000 ml or more within the same timeframe' (World Health Organization (WHO) 2012: 8; Mavrides et al 2016). It has also been defined using the context of adversely affecting 'maternal physiology, such as blood pressure and hematocrit' (ICD-10 2018). Primary PPH occurs within 24 hours of the birth, and secondary PPH occurs after 24 hours and up to 6 weeks after the birth (Alexander et al 2002). However, when describing PPH, it is important to take into account the fact that blood loss is notoriously difficult to estimate accurately, and that any significant blood loss in a previously anaemic woman could result in considerable morbidity (Moore & Chandraharan 2010).

Consequences

The recent report on maternal deaths in the UK by Knight et al (2017) revealed an increase in the number of women who had died from catastrophic haemorrhage since the previous triennial report, from 17 to 22. Of these, 9 deaths were from an atonic uterus, 5 of these following a caesarean birth, and 1 related to genital tract trauma. PPH is the second highest cause of maternal death in the UK, preceded by thrombosis or thromboembolism. Globally, however, PPH is the most common cause of maternal death, particularly in low-income countries (WHO 2012), thought to be up to one in four maternal deaths (Carroll et al 2016).

Such catastrophic haemorrhage is a major concern, but even moderate haemorrhage can have a significant impact on a woman's experience of motherhood, with the potential for fatigue, lethargy, failure to breastfeed and the need for medication or blood transfusion (El-Refaey & Rodeck 2003). In addition, some evidence points to the detrimental effects on the physical and psychological well-being of women (Carroll et al 2016) as well as a lower number of women conceiving a pregnancy after experiencing PPH following a caesarean section (Fullerton et al 2013).

Postnatal observation

After the birth, irrespective of the mode, the midwife must monitor the woman's condition to assess whether her recovery remains within normal parameters. In the immediate hours after the birth, part of the midwife's observations will include assessment of the woman's blood loss and uterine tone. Measurement of blood pressure, temperature and heart rate are also key elements of the initial postnatal examination, and should be re-employed if the woman's blood loss increases. In addition, respiration rate should be monitored, as breathlessness is a symptom of anaemia. It should be noted that in some cases the development of maternal tachycardia and hypotension may not occur immediately (Abdul-kadir et al 2014). All observations should be recorded on a Modified Early Obstetric Warning System (MEOWS) chart and escalated as required.

Estimation of blood loss

It is acknowledged that the amount of blood a woman loses after birth is extremely difficult to estimate, particularly when the loss is either very small or very large (Razvi et al 1996). One study concluded that midwives and obstetricians visually underestimated blood loss by 40% to 49% (Maslovitz et al 2008). Another study has demonstrated that student midwives are more likely to underestimate the quantity of blood loss than qualified midwives and use of an online training tool was recommended (Pranal et al 2018).

A review of the studies aiming to improve identification of PPH highlighted that so far, studies have tended to focus on improving estimates of blood loss by volume (Hancock et al 2015). They argue that decision making around PPH, however, relates to the observations of the speed and type of blood loss as well as the physical condition of the woman.

Alternative methods to estimation are more quantitative, by comparing the dry and blood-stained weights of the materials used around the birth area (for example, Jones 2015). This may be an effective method within a clinical hospital setting, but more complex when the blood loss occurs in a water birth or a home environment.

Activity

Access the paper by Brant (1967). Identify the issues relating to estimation of blood loss highlighted historically and consider the similarities and differences in practice 50 years later.

Find out the methods for estimating blood loss in your area.

How do clinicians practise estimating blood loss in your area? Create an opportunity for practising this.

Predisposing antenatal factors

It is known that certain women are more at risk for PPH than others. The risk factors that are avoidable, such as anaemia, should be identified and treated, especially if another known risk factor is also likely, such as caesarean birth.

Box 6.1 lists the factors in the antenatal period that may lead to PPH.

Activity

Consider the list of potential antenatal predisposing factors for PPH alongside your knowledge of anatomy and physiology. Try and work out why each of the factors on the list may lead to PPH.

Box 6.1 **Potential antenatal factors leading to postpartum haemorrhage**

- Nulliparity
- Maternal BMI of more than 35% to 50% higher risk
- Macrosomia
- Multiple pregnancy/polyhydramnios
- Antepartum haemorrhage
- Previous PPH (risk recurrence 8%–10%)
- Pre-eclampsia/raised BP
- Previous C/S (placenta previa)
- Asian/Hispanic descent
- Anaemia < 9 g/dl
- Fibroids

Table 6.1: **The 4 Ts: causes of postpartum haemorrhage**

4 Ts	Causes
Tone	Relaxed or atonic uterus, bleeding from the placental site
Trauma	Episiotomy or lacerations to the cervix or vagina; inverted or ruptured uterus, pelvic haematoma
Tissue	Retained placental tissue or fragment of membrane
Thrombin	Coagulopathy

Causes of PPH

Excessive blood loss originates from one of four sources often called 'The 4 Ts' (see Table 6.1). Globally, the main cause of PPH relates to the 'tone' of the uterus: lack of efficient uterine contraction (WHO 2012), which could be in the region of 63% of severe bleeding (Nyfløt et al 2017). In the same study 'trauma' accounted for 18%, 'tissue' causes for 36% and 'thrombin' for 1.5%.

Tone

Uterine tone can be compromised in a number of ways. If the uterus has been over-extended because of a multiple gestation, macrosomia or poly-hydramnios, its ability to contract effectively may be reduced. Also, if the uterine muscle has been overworked after a rapid or prolonged labour or in cases of grand multiparity, its tone will be impaired. Tone might also be reduced in the presence of an intra-amniotic infection or if the uterus has a structural anomaly such as septum or uterine fibroids.

It is also important to remember that the uterus may not contract effectively if the woman has a very full bladder. The use of a fifth 'T' for 'Toilet' will help in remembering that this may be an important factor to resolve.

Trauma

Women who have had an instrumental or precipitous birth are more at risk of PPH after lacerations to the perineum, vagina or cervix. Previous caesarean birth or any uterine surgery creates an increased risk of uterine rupture and severe internal bleeding.

Tissue

If there are any remnants of tissue inside the uterus after the birth, they impair its ability to contract effectively. If the placenta and membranes were incomplete at the end of labour, or the placenta was adherent, it is possible that fragments could remain in the uterine cavity, leading to severe haemorrhage.

Activity

Find out about
- von Willebrand's syndrome and the effect on pregnancy
- HELLP syndrome
- DIC
  Consider why these situations could lead to PPH.

Thrombin

Abnormalities of coagulation can result from a range of sources. The woman may have a history of previous coagulopathy and have been treated with anti-coagulation therapy during her pregnancy. She may have a pre-existing condition such as von Willebrand's syndrome (Demers et al 2005). If she has had pre-eclampsia, her platelet count may have decreased (thrombocytopenia). HELLP syndrome (hemolysis, elevated liver enzymes and low platelet count) will also have an impact on blood factors that could impact clotting. Other events in pregnancy such as amniotic fluid embolism, antepartum haemorrhage or intrauterine death may have increased the woman's risk of developing disseminated intravascular coagulation (DIC), ultimately impairing the blood's ability to clot.

Prevention of PPH

Activity

Review your knowledge of the expectant or physiological management and the active management of the third stage of labour.

Look at your local guidelines for labour and compare to the National Institute for Health and Care Excellence (NICE) guidelines (2014, 2017) for care in the third stage.

In a systematic review of the evidence it was identified that active management of the third stage of labour versus expectant management significantly reduces the risk of PPH of greater than 1000 ml, though this is not significant for women with lower risk (Begley et al 2015). In most labour wards in acute hospital settings it is usual practice to offer an oxytocic drug to be administered to the woman, with her consent, via an intramuscular injection in her leg after delivery of the baby's anterior shoulder. (For further information and discussion about the management of the third stage and women's choice see Baston & Hall 2017). For active management of the third stage of labour, NICE (2017) recommends the use of 10 IU by intramuscular injection. A combination of ergometrine and oxytocin is associated with more vomiting and an increase in blood pressure than syntocinon alone, with little added value to preventing minor PPH in women who are at low risk. However, a combined oxytocin–syntocinon product is advocated when a woman is known to be high risk of PPH and normotensive (Mavrides et al 2016).

As oxytocics should be stored in the dark in a refrigerator, and must be administered via sterile needle and syringe by a person with the technical skill, it would not be an appropriate means of preventing PPH in many low-income countries. Misoprostol is the recommended drug of choice in these countries, as it is an inexpensive option and does not need refrigeration (Begley et al 2015).

The use of misoprostol is associated with several side effects that are both dose and route related. Shivering and pyrexia are associated with its use even at low doses, and their incidence increases with increased doses. Higher doses are also associated with gastrointestinal disturbances, including nausea, vomiting and diarrhoea. The incidence of side effects is lower when misoprostol is given rectally rather than orally (Gulmezoglu et al 2004).

Activity

- Which oxytocic drugs are used for the active management of the third stage of labour where you work? When is ergometrine contraindicated?
- Is a physiological third stage of labour offered to women where you work?
- Find out about the drugs carboprost and carbetocin.

A large randomized trial of administration of the drug antifibrinolytic tranexamic acid (1 g IV for women who were diagnosed with a PPH) within 3 hours of birth demonstrated that this drug is effective in preventing deaths from PPH (WOMAN trial collaborators 2017). As this is currently available only in intravenous form it would not be suitable for women in many low-income countries (Shakur et al 2018). More research is needed into the use of this drug more widely.

Diagnosis

+   **Vaginal blood loss** In most cases excessive blood loss will be visible – either in the pool or, if the woman gave birth on a mattress, soaking through the sanitary pad, clothing and bedding. In some women, blood loss is concealed in a haematoma, in the pelvic cavity or in a relaxed uterus. A uterus that has filled with blood, lacks tone and becomes broad is said to feel 'boggy' or 'spongy' on abdominal palpation.
+   **Deterioration in maternal well-being** In severe cases the woman may lose consciousness and collapse. Her symptoms will depend on the degree of blood loss and her pre-birth health status. Most women, however, will not experience severe cardiovascular changes with a blood loss of between 500 and 1000 ml, but further loss will result in increased heart rate, falling blood pressure, pallor, agitation and dizziness. In severe cases, where blood loss is 2000 to 3000 ml, the woman will stop passing urine and develop air hunger, the signs of shock.

Care and treatment

Guidelines

The most recent triennial report on maternal deaths (Knight et al 2017) highlights particular aspects of concern around care:

+   There should not be reliance on one haemaglobin blood test result that has been reassuring and resuscitation fluids should be started as soon as possible.
+   There should be extreme caution on the use of misoprostol when a woman has had a late intrauterine fetal death, especially if she also has a uterine scar.
+   If a woman is showing signs of hypovolaemic shock (tachycardia and/or agitation and the late sign of hypotension) concealed haemorrhage should be considered even where no bleeding is noted externally.
+   Ongoing careful observation and support should be made of women who have had a serious haemorrhage and escalation of care when there is continued bleeding or clinical concerns (a massive haemorrhage call activated).

The report also raises concerns about appropriate staffing for units as women are more at risk of serious events where this has not been in place.

Care for women with PPH

As with other situations in this book, any care for women with PPH must be carried out in the context of the multi-disciplinary team and include appropriate referral to other health professionals (Nursing and Midwifery Council (NMC) 2017). The NMC standards also expect that a midwife will:

> *'use skills in managing obstetric and neonatal emergencies, under-pinned by appropriate knowledge' (NMC 2017: 4)*

A PPH may occur at any time, including in a home birth setting. Therefore a midwife should be able to provide initial emergency care in the circumstances of a PPH until help arrives and to continue the care alongside the other members of the team. At all times care of the woman should promote her dignity and wellbeing and communication should be appropriate to her and her birthing partner, as it will be a stressful and alarming situation (Mavrides et al 2016). For a flow chart of actions after identification of PPH see Fig. 6.1.

Immediate action

1. Call for help

In the event of a primary PPH at home, the midwife should ask the woman's partner or second midwife to dial the emergency number (999 in the UK) and ask for a paramedic ambulance. If the woman is in hospital, the woman's birth partner can be asked to pull the emergency buzzer (systems vary between hospitals), which will bring a colleague who can summon appropriate medical assistance. The Midwives' Standards of competence (NMC 2017: 4) state that in an emergency the midwife should 'access appropriate assistance'. This means that in the event of a life-threatening PPH, for example, the midwife should call a professional who can make a significant contribution to the woman's wellbeing, such as a senior obstetrician. The senior midwife coordinating the labour ward would be well placed to organize the activity.

2. Stop the bleeding

Initial management of PPH will focus on stabilizing the woman's condition and controlling the bleeding. However, when the midwife discovers a woman

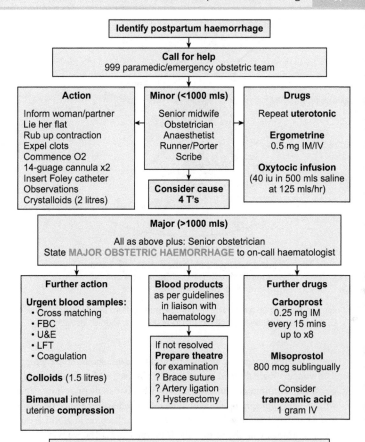

Fig. 6.1 Action for care of a woman with postpartum haemorrhage.

who is bleeding heavily, during her initial resuscitative measures she should be trying to identify precisely where the bleeding originates. As an atonic uterus is the most likely cause, she should start by locating the uterus abdominally.

'Tone' as a cause of haemorrhage

The uterus should be very firm, central and contracted. If it feels soft and broad the fundus should be massaged with a circular motion; this activity is known as 'rubbing up a contraction' (see Fig. 6.2). The uterus should

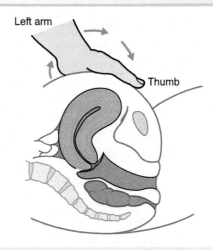

Left arm

Thumb

The left hand is cupped over the uterus ( ) and massages it with a firm circular motion in a clockwise direction

Fig. 6.2 Rubbing up a contraction. (With permission from Macdonald S, Johnson G, eds., Mayes Midwifery, 15th ed., p. 1094, Fig. 67.2. Oxford: Elsevier.)

respond by becoming firm, at which point the midwife should stop rubbing. The woman's vaginal blood loss should be observed while simultaneously giving her a running commentary about what her midwife is doing and why. Where appropriate, she should be told who has come into the room and what they are doing. It takes no extra time to keep smiling, which can give the woman confidence that she is in safe hands. The woman's birth partner will also need reassurance, and he or she should be encouraged to sit down, as many people faint unexpectedly at the sight of blood. If the uterus does not contract it is possible the woman has a full bladder which is preventing this. If she is not able to pass urine normally in a bed pan, providing the woman has given informed consent, a short catheter may be passed and the bladder emptied, which may solve the problem of bleeding. However, if bleeding is rapid an indwelling catheter should be passed, as it will be important to measure fluid balance (see Chapter 1: Maternal collapse).

3. Give a uterotonic drug

If the blood loss was anything more than a short gush that stopped as soon as the uterus contracted again, an oxytocic drug should be administered.

If the woman had consented to the active management of the third stage of labour, she will already have received oxytocin 10 units IM when the baby's anterior shoulder was delivered (NICE 2014, 2017). If the woman had a PPH after a physiological third stage, she should be offered oxytocic drugs at this stage following explanation. The uterotonic drug may be repeated or give ergometrine 500 mcg IM up to a maximum dose of 1 mg (2 doses).

> ## Activity
> Find the guidance for caring for women with PPH in your area of work and learn the protocol of the drug regime. Find out where emergency medication is stored and what drugs community-based midwives carry.

If the bleeding does not respond to oxytocin or ergometrine, then 250 micrograms of the prostaglandin carboprost should be given IM or directly into the myometrium by a doctor. The doses can be repeated, at least 15 minutes apart, up to a maximum dose of 2 milligrams.

This may now be followed by the use of tranexamic acid, as explained previously.

Bi-manual uterine compression

If bleeding continues, bi-manual uterine compression should be employed to reduce any further loss (see Fig. 6.3). This emergency procedure involves the midwife inserting her dominant hand (made into a fist) into the woman's vagina, aiming for the anterior fornix. Abdominally, using her other hand, she then compresses the posterior wall of the uterus against her vaginal fist. The compression is maintained until the bleeding stops and the uterus contracts.

> ## Activity
> Reflect on the anatomy and physiology that underpins the use of bi-manual uterine compression.

4. Resuscitate the woman

It is important to read this section alongside the information provided in Chapter 1 regarding care of the collapsed woman.

In minor PPH, one wide-bore cannulae should be sited (antecubital fossa) and fluid replaced with normal saline or other crystalloids. When there is more severe bleeding two intravenous infusions should be sited.

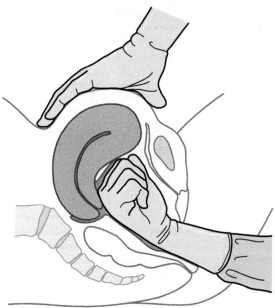

Fig. 6.3 Internal bi-manual compression of the uterus. (With permission from Macdonald S, Johnson G, eds., Mayes Midwifery, 15th ed., p. 1097, Fig. 67.3. Oxford: Elsevier.)

A continuous infusion of fluid including a uterotonic is recommended and in the UK 40 units of syntocinon are combined with a 500 ml of fluid at 125 ml/hour (Mavrides et al 2016).

Extreme caution should be observed and close monitoring of fluid balance maintained when administering oxytocin infusions – especially if one had been used during labour – owing to the risk of water intoxication. A MEOWS chart would be used. In cases of severe PPH, a urinary catheter should be inserted and the output of urine monitored meticulously. For severe case of PPH an arterial line may be required with a potential transfer to an intensive therapy unit.

Surgical interventions

If the woman continues to bleed despite the use of uterotonic agents and application of pressure, she is at risk of developing clotting problems that will further exacerbate the problem. Potential interventions that may take place are listed in the activity box that follows.

To save a woman's life, as a final resort it may be necessary for her to undergo a total abdominal hysterectomy. This will be a shocking situation for her and her partner and the midwife should be aware of the potential psychological impact.

'Tissue' as a cause of haemorrhage

If the placenta is still in situ and an oxytocic drug has been given, attempts should be made to deliver it by controlled cord traction. A full bladder can impede uterine contraction and should be emptied. If the placenta remains undelivered, attempts should be made to remove it manually. A doctor should perform this procedure, often in a theatre environment, under anaesthetic, with an intravenous infusion in progress.

Manual removal of the placenta by a midwife

In very rare circumstances a midwife would need to undertake manual removal of the placenta. The Standards for competence for registered midwives (NMC 2017: 7) state that midwives should be able to:

'Undertake appropriate emergency procedures to meet the health needs of women and babies.'

This will include emergency procedures such as manual removal of the placenta and manual examination of the uterus. Most midwives practising in the UK will never find themselves in circumstances in which they need to exercise this skill. It is, however, a procedure they should understand, not only because they might need to act in an emergency but also because they will be faced with situations in which they need to support women undergoing manual removal of the placenta and their medical colleagues performing it.

If nitrous oxide is available, the woman should be encouraged to use it. The midwife inserts her coned dominant hand into the woman's vagina. By following the cord, the placenta is located and a separated edge identified. The fingers are gently inserted between the placenta and the uterine wall (the cleavage plane) with the back of the hand against the uterus. The non-dominant hand supports the uterine fundus abdominally while the midwife employs a gentle side-to-side movement with her vaginal hand to peel the placenta from the uterine wall. Once entirely separated, a contraction should be 'rubbed up' using the non-dominant hand and the placenta removed from the uterus. The placenta should then be examined for completeness.

'Trauma' as a cause of blood loss

If, on initial assessment of uterine tone, the uterus is found to be well contracted, the next most likely source of bleeding is trauma to the genital tract. Gentle exploration of the perineum should begin and pressure applied with a sterile pack to the bleeding site while another midwife prepares for prompt suturing of the wound. If a specific bleeding vessel can be identified, sterile artery forceps can be applied to it directly. If an episiotomy had been performed, this should be repaired without delay. Labial and clitoral tears can also be a source of significant blood loss, requiring immediate repair. If bleeding continues, despite no obvious external trauma, uterine rupture may be the cause, requiring rapid surgical intervention.

Activity
What are the signs and symptoms of uterine inversion?
How should this condition be treated?
How would a pelvic haematoma be recognized and treated?

'Thrombin' as a cause of blood loss

Coagulopathy should be suspected if the blood that is lost does not clot. The woman will require blood products to replace clotting factors as well as further treatment specific to her condition. Her care should be managed in consultation with a haematologist (Mavrides et al 2016), and once her condition is stabilized she should be cared for in a high-dependency or intensive care environment.

Secondary PPH

Occurring at least 24 hours after the birth and before 12 weeks (Alexander et al 2002), secondary PPH can come as a severe shock to the woman. It may result from retained placental fragments, infection such as endometriosis or, rarely, an unsecured blood vessel after caesarean birth or ruptured uterine artery (Chandraharan & Krishna 2017). Although secondary PPH is generally associated with morbidity rather than mortality, blood loss can be just as catastrophic as with a primary postpartum haemorrhage and requires the same immediate response. If the woman is at home, and bleeding is severe, a paramedic ambulance should be summoned and an intravenous infusion started before transfer to an obstetric unit.

If there are retained products of conception, ultrasound may be used, though the diagnosis is thought to be unreliable (Mavrides et al 2016). In many cases examination of the uterus under anaesthetic is the only means of identifying the source of the bleeding. It is also recommended that high vaginal and endocervical swabs should be taken for suspected endometritis and antibiotic therapy commenced (Mavrides et al 2016). Once the cause of the haemorrhage has been treated, the woman should be observed for signs of subsequent infection and anaemia.

REFLECTION ON THE TRIGGER SCENARIO

Look back at the trigger scenario:

> Debra is holding her new baby skin-to-skin after birth. She starts to shift uncomfortably in the bed. She turns to Emily, the midwife, and says, 'I feel really wet'.

Now that you are familiar with the principles of PPH you should have some insight into the evidence and how the scenario relates to it. The jigsaw model will be used to explore the scenario in more depth.

Effective communication

Appropriate and effective communication is expected as an important part of a midwife's role (NMC 2017). This will include communication with the woman and her family as well as appropriate referral to other members of the multi-professional team. In this scenario the midwife, Emily, needs to observe, ask important questions to establish what level of action should be taken and employ effective listening skills. Questions that could be asked are: What key questions will she ask Debra about her feelings and symptoms? How will she ask her to show her why she is 'wet'? How will she contact immediate help and who will she ask to help her? How will she communicate to the multi-disciplinary team what is taking place? Where will she record her actions?

Woman-centred care

It is expected that a woman should be central to her care and that she should have an informed choice around the decisions related to her care even within a complicated situation. Questions that could be asked are: How can Emily ensure that Debra is central to the actions she will take?

How will she invite Debra to reveal the cause for the 'wet' and continue to promote her dignity and wellbeing? How will Emily ensure Debra has choice in this circumstance? How will the well-being of the mother–baby dyad be promoted and maintained in this situation?

Using best evidence

In this circumstance, it is important to be aware what the best evidence is surrounding the care of women after the birth of a baby. Which care setting does the evidence relate to? Questions that could be asked are: Could this PPH have been anticipated or prevented? What is known about the risk factors that may have put Debra at risk of a PPH? What is the evidence surrounding the treatment of a PPH? What are the side effects of ergometrine? What is the best way to determine blood loss after a birth? Are there any research studies currently looking at the best way to treat PPH?

Professional and legal issues

At all times, the midwife should act professionally within her scope of practice (NMC 2017) and according to the law. She also has a duty to her employer to fulfil the requirements of her profession. Questions that could be asked are: What is Emily's responsibility as a midwife regarding complex care situations? How will she ensure she is acting within the Code of Practice (NMC 2015) in relation to involving other members of the care team? What is her duty of care regarding Debra's baby and her partner? What is the law regarding obtaining Debra's informed consent regarding choices about her care?

Team working

In most situations in midwifery practice midwives do not work in isolation but are part of a wider multi-disciplinary team. Midwives who work in the community setting are often working autonomously and will have specific lines of escalation to follow when they require support in an emergency. Within a hospital birth unit, a midwife works within a team of colleagues and usually has senior midwifery and medical staff to call on when needed. However, wherever a midwife works, she must be able to provide initial care and treatment, until further assistance becomes available. Questions that could be asked are: Who are the members of the multi-disciplinary team? Who should be informed about Debra's condition? Why should Emily tell them and how? If this is a complex circumstance, who is responsible for Debra's care? Has the team undertaken multi-professional training for this situation? What is the role of the student midwife in PPH?

Clinical dexterity

In this situation Emily may need clinical dexterity to assess and deal with a serious condition. Her skills and competence will have built up over time and in response to her exposure to such situations previously and regular skills and drills training. Questions that could be asked are: In this scenario what are Emily's clinical responsibilities? What observations should be carried out? How will she carry these out while maintaining Debra's dignity and well-being? What physical examinations should be carried out by Emily? What physical emergency care will she carry out? Has she had appropriate training to complete emergency care? How will Emily maintain her skills?

Models of care

There are many of models of care practised and each of these will present advantages and disadvantages in relation to caring for a woman experiencing PPH. Questions that may be asked are: In this situation has Debra had her birth at home, birth centre or hospital unit? Has Emily been the midwife responsible for the birth? Who will be the lead professional for this circumstance? Who else is available to summon and provide help? What models of care are available where you work and how does the emergency response differ for each of these?

Safe environment

At all times consideration should be made of the most appropriate environment for care of the woman and her baby. Whether this scenario was in a home, birth centre or hospital a decision will need to be made regarding where Debra would be safest. Questions that may be asked are: Where is the safest environment for Debra to be? How will Emily create the safest environment for her and her baby? If Debra needs urgent assistance at home, who should Emily contact? What equipment will Emily have to support a swift and appropriate response to an emergency situation at home? How will Emily support the safe care of Debra's baby during any emergency treatment?

Promotes health

The aim of all care is to promote the well-being of the woman and her baby. This will include her emotional, spiritual and social health as well as her physical needs. Questions that may be asked are: How will Emily promote Debra's whole well-being during this circumstance? How may she help alleviate any anxieties she or her partner may have? After the management and treatment of the emergency situation, what other considerations should be taken into account to ensure that Debra is able to continue motherhood in the best physical and emotional health?

Further scenarios

SCENARIO 1

A locum doctor has just carried out a ventouse birth for a baby where the labour was delayed. The baby is lying skin-to-skin with the woman. A uterotonic drug was administered with the birth of the baby. Caroline, the midwife, notes the doctor is pulling forcefully on the umbilical cord and that the woman cries in pain.

Practice point

It is possible that midwives will work with members of the team who have not had appropriate training regarding birth. They may need to advise others to prevent serious events taking place. In this situation use of force, where a placenta remains adherent for whatever reason, may result in uterine inversion.

- How will Caroline respond to this situation to advocate for the woman concerned?
- What will she say to the doctor?
- What are the priorities of care in the situation?
- Who may be called from the multidisciplinary team to help?
- What is the immediate care required should a uterine inversion take place?
- How may an adherent placenta be diagnosed and treated?
- How will this situation be documented?

SCENARIO 2

Verity is transferred home after a caesarean section. On the seventh day after the birth Sandy, the midwife, receives a telephone call from James, Verity's partner, saying that they were worried as Verity seemed to have passed a large clot on her pad and was bleeding fresh red blood again.

Practice point

Midwives are often the first point of contact for emergency calls in the community setting. Women who have had caesarean sections are more likely to develop infections after their operations, but there may be other reasons for the development of bleeding again, such as increased activity.

- What questions will Sandy ask James?
- Will Sandy need to speak to Verity?

- How will she assess the cause of the bleeding?
- What will she advise Verity to do?
- Will she go and visit at home or suggest Verity attend hospital?
- What observations will be made?
- What treatment may be required?

Conclusion

PPH is a major source of morbidity and mortality for childbearing women around the world. Prompt action by the midwife can help minimize the impact of this traumatic event along with rapid support from members of the multi-disciplinary team. Local guidelines should reflect recent advances in knowledge and algorithms of care developed nationally, and teams should practise what to do about this emergency on a regular basis to save women's lives.

Resources

Pranal, M., Guttman, A., Ouchchane, L., et al. 2018. Visual estimation of blood loss. Available at: http://www.audipog.net/estimated-loss.html

Drug use and side effects: British National Formulary
https://bnf.nice.org.uk/drug/ergometrine-maleate.html#indicationsAndDoses

Impact of simulation training for PPH
Egenberg, S., Øian, P., Eggebø, T., et al., 2017. Changes in self-efficacy, collective efficacy and patient outcome after interprofessional simulation training on postpartum haemorrhage. J. Clin. Nurs. 26, 3174–3187.

Blood transfusion information for women
https://www.nhs.uk/conditions/blood-transfusion/

NHS blood transfusion and transplant
https://www.nhsbt.nhs.uk/what-we-do/blood-services/blood-transfusion/

Infographic diagnosis and management of postpartum haemorrhage
BMJ 2017; 358. Available at: http://www.bmj.com/content/bmj/suppl/2017/09/27/bmj.j3875.DC1/chae036081.wi.pdf

References

Abdul-Kadir, R., McLintock, C., Ducloy, A.S., et al., 2014. Evaluation and management of postpartum haemorrhage: consensus from an international expert panel. Transfusion 54, 1756–1768.

Alexander, J., Thomas, P., Sanghera, J., 2002. Treatments for secondary postpartum haemorrhage. Cochrane Database Syst. Rev. (1), No: CD002867, doi:10.1002/14651858.CD002867.

Baston, H., Hall, J., 2017. Midwifery Essentials: Labour, vol. 3. Elsevier, Oxford.

Begley, C.M., Gyte, G.M.L., Devane, D., et al., 2015. Active versus expectant management for women in the third stage of labour. Cochrane Database Syst. Rev. (3), CD007412, doi:10.1002/14651858.CD007412.pub4.

Brant, H., 1967. Precise estimation of postpartum haemorrhage: difficulties and importance. Br. Med. J. 18, 398–400.

Briley, A., Seed, P., Tydeman, G., et al., 2014. Reporting errors, incidence and risk factors for postpartum haemorrhage and progression to severe PPH: a prospective observational study. BJOG 121, 876–888.

Carroll, M., Daly, D., Begley, C.M., 2016. The prevalence of women's emotional and physical health problems following a postpartum haemorrhage: a systematic review. BMC Pregnancy Childbirth 16, 261. https://doi.org/10.1186/s12884-016-1054-1.

Chandraharan, E., Krishna, A., 2017. Diagnosis and management of postpartum haemorrhage. BMJ 358, j3875.

Demers, C., Derzko, C., David, M., et al., 2005. Gynaecological and obstetric management of women with inherited bleeding disorders. J. Obstet. Gynaecol. Can. 27, 707–732.

El-Refaey, H., Rodeck, C., 2003. Post-partum haemorrhage: definitions, medical and surgical management. A time for change. Br. Med. Bull. 67, 205–217.

Fullerton, G., Danielian, P., Bhattacharya, S., 2013. Outcomes of pregnancy following postpartum haemorrhage. BJOG 120, 621–627.

Gulmezoglu, A., Forna, F., Villar, J., Hofmeyr, G., 2004. Prostaglandins for the prevention of postpartum haemorrhage. Cochrane Database Syst. Rev. (1), CD000494. pub2. doi:10.1002/14651858.CD000494.pub2.

Hancock, A., Weeks, A.D., Lavender, D.T., 2015. Is accurate and reliable blood loss estimation the 'crucial step' in early detection of postpartum haemorrhage: an integrative review of the literature. BMC Pregnancy Childbirth 15, 230.

ICD-10, 2018. ICD-10-CM diagnosis code. Available at: http://www.icd10data.com/ICD10CM/Codes/O00-O9A/O60-O77/O72-.

Jones, R., 2015. Quantitative measurement of blood loss during delivery. JOGNN 44 (s1), s41.

Knight, M., Paterson-Brown, S., on behalf of the haemorrhage and AFE chapter-writing group, 2017. Messages for care of women with haemorrhage or amniotic fluid embolism. In: Knight, M, Nair M, Tuffnell D, et al, eds., Saving Lives, Improving Mothers' Care Lessons Learned to Inform Maternity Care from the UK and Ireland Confidential Enquiries into Maternal Deaths and Morbidity 2013–15. Available at: https://www.npeu.ox.ac.uk/downloads/files/mbrrace-uk/reports/MBRRACE-UK%20Maternal%20Report%202017%20-%20Web.pdf.

Maslovitz, S., Barkai, G., Lessing, J.B., et al., 2008. Improved accuracy of postpartum blood loss estimation as assessed by simulation. Acta Obstet. Gynecol. Scand. 87, 929–934.

Mavrides, E., Allard, S., Chandraharan, E., et al. on behalf of the Royal College of Obstetricians and Gynaecologists, 2016. Prevention and management of postpartum haemorrhage. BJOG 124, e106–e149. Available at: http://onlinelibrary.wiley.com/doi/10.1111/1471-0528.14178/epdf.

Moore, J., Chandraharan, E., 2010. Management of massive postpartum haemorrhage and coagulopathy. Obstet Gynaecol Reprod Med 20, 174–180.

National Institute for Health and Care Excellence (NICE), 2014. updated 2017 Intrapartum care: care for healthy women and babies. NICE CG190. Available at: https://www.nice.org.uk/guidance/cg190.

NMC, 2015. The Code: Standards of Conduct, Performance, and Ethics for Nurses and Midwives. Nursing and Midwifery Council, London.

Nursing and Midwifery Council (NMC), 2017. Standards for competence for registered midwives. Available at: https://www.nmc.org.uk/globalassets/sitedocuments/standards/nmc-standards-for-competence-for-registered-midwives.pdf.

Nyfløt, L.T., Sandven, I., Stray-Pedersen, B., et al., 2017. Risk factors for severe postpartum hemorrhage: a case-control study. BMC Pregnancy Childbirth 17, 17.

Oberg, A.S., Hernandez-Diaz, S., Palmsten, K., et al., 2014. Patterns of recurrence of postpartum hemorrhage in a large population-based cohort. Am. J. Obstet. Gynecol. 210 (3), 229.e1–229.e8.

Pranal, M., Guttmann, A., Ouchchane, L., et al., 2018. Do estimates of blood loss differ between student midwives and midwives? A multicenter cross-sectional study. Midwifery 59, 17–22.

Razvi, K., Chua, S., Arulkumaran, S., Ratnam, S., 1996. A comparison between visual estimation and laboratory determination of blood loss during the third stage of labour. Aust. N. Z. J. Obstet. Gynaecol. 36 (2), 152–154.

Shakur, H., Beaumont, D., Pavord, S., et al., 2018. Antifibrinolytic drugs for treating primary postpartum haemorrhage. Cochrane Database Syst. Rev. (2), CD012964, doi:10.1002/14651858.CD012964.

WOMAN trial collaborators, 2017. Effect of early tranexamic acid administration on mortality, hysterectomy, and other morbidities in women with post-partum haemorrhage (WOMAN): an international, randomised, double-blind, placebo-controlled trial. Lancet 389 (10084), 2105–2116.

WHO, 2012. WHO recommendations for the prevention and treatment of post-partum haemorrhage. World Health Organization, Geneva. Available at: http://apps.who.int/iris/bitstream/10665/75411/1/9789241548502_eng.pdf?ua=1.

CHAPTER 7

Eclampsia

TRIGGER SCENARIO

Keira gave birth to her first baby an hour and a half ago. She suddenly says, 'My eyes have gone blurred and I feel dizzy'. She collapses, and Val, the midwife caring for her, sees she has noticeable convulsive movements of her body.

Introduction

Eclampsia is a rare condition in the UK that may be experienced in a large maternity unit on average only once a year. It is therefore possible that a midwife may never care for a woman with this condition in the UK, although those intending to work abroad may see the condition more frequently (Roberts et al 2011). Furthermore, it may occur more frequently in women who have been displaced from other cultures and are unable to communicate their needs.

Its serious nature means that a midwife must know what causes eclampsia, how to recognize its onset and how it may be treated, to limit its potential impact.

Eclampsia is a condition that causes women to experience one or more convulsions similar to an epileptic fit during pregnancy, labour or postnatally. It is usually, but not always, following presentation of pre-eclampsia (Bothamley & Boyle 2017).

Activity

- Review the physiology of blood pressure in pregnancy.
- What are the clinical signs and symptoms of the condition pre-eclampsia?

Symptoms of eclampsia

The convulsions of eclampsia are tonic–clonic seizures thought to be caused by cerebral vasospasm which leads to ischaemia in that part of the woman's brain and 'disruption' to the blood–brain barrier and oedema. Magnetic resonance imaging (MRI) has demonstrated blood flow in the cerebral artery is increased in women with pre-eclampsia, which is thought may be a precursor to eclampsia (Zeeman et al 2004). Other conditions may cause seizures as well, and these may need to be excluded.

Presentation of such seizures is an obstetric emergency and demands immediate medical assistance, according to the Standards for Midwifery practice (Nursing and Midwifery Council (NMC) 2017).

> **Activity**
>
> Describe the signs and symptoms of tonic–clonic and absence seizures.

Incidence of eclampsia

Eclampsia is a rare condition in the UK, reported to be around 2.7 cases per 10000 births (Knight 2007). Globally, however, it is estimated that 14% of women die as a result of eclampsia, although it is more prevalent in developing countries (Say et al 2014). Over time deaths from hypertensive conditions and eclampsia have been reducing in the UK and only two women have died as a result in recent years (Knight et al 2016).

An eclamptic seizure can occur in the second half of pregnancy, during labour or postnatally. The incidence in the antepartum period has been reported at 71% versus 29% postpartum (Shenone et al 2013). The condition may be more serious if it occurs in the antenatal period; it may result in more complications for the mother and has a higher neonatal mortality rate, usually as a result of the infant being preterm (Douglas & Redman 1994). Therefore vigilance is required for those women who present with pre-eclampsia early in pregnancy.

A large, multicentre randomized trial on whether to treat severe pre-eclampsia with the anticonvulsant drug magnesium sulphate before the onset of eclampsia was carried out between 1998 and 2001 (Magpie Trial Collaborative Group 2002). The women included in the trial had either yet to give birth or were in the first 24 hours postnatal; they had had blood pressure readings of 90 mm Hg diastolic or 140 mm Hg systolic or more on at least two occasions; proteinuria was 1 + or more; and practitioners were uncertain about whether to use magnesium sulphate. This study showed that the use of magnesium sulphate reduced the onset of eclampsia by half. Since its introduction as the treatment of choice, maternal deaths in the UK have diminished (Duley et al 2010a).

Risk factors

Eclampsia appears to occur more in women who are experiencing their first pregnancies. Predisposing factors are suggested to be previous chronic hypertension, diabetes, obesity, certain ethnicities and low socioeconomic status (Steegers et al 2010). However, as with pre-eclampsia, it is wise to be aware of those women whose subsequent pregnancies result from new relationships, as this may constitute a potential risk factor. It is suggested that there may be some climactic factors that could lead to an increased chance of eclampsia (Subramaniam 2007).

The rare nature of this condition means that there is a lack of statistical evidence on its management, especially in relation to morbidity. However, in an assessment of cases in the UK it was noted that those who experienced recurrent fits were more likely to be preterm (Knight 2007). The changes in treatment in recent years have resulted in fewer cases. It was noted in the same study that 63% of the women who had eclampsia had not previously had signs of serious pre-eclampsia (Knight et al 2007). Globally, eclampsia appears to occur more in women in low-resourced areas with lack of access to effective medical support in pregnancy (Bellizzi et al 2017).

Warning signs and symptoms

The only 'sign' of eclampsia is convulsions in the mother. However, the association with pre-eclampsia is indicated by the name. Symptoms relating to hypertension, proteinuria and oedema are not present in all women (Knight 2007), which means that currently, though it may be possible to predict pre-eclampsia (Poon & Nicolaides 2014), the ability to predict the onset of eclampsia is difficult, despite women receiving regular antenatal care.

However, in an earlier study more than half of the women experienced extreme symptoms, which included headaches (50%), visual disturbance (19%) or epigastric pain (19%) before the seizure (Douglas & Redman 1994). In Knight's (2007) study 79% had at least one symptom in the week before the fit: headaches (56%), hypertension with diastolic greater than 90 mm Hg (48%), proteinuria of 1 + or more on dipstick of greater than 0.3 gram in 24 hours (46%), both hypertension and proteinuria (38%), visual disturbance (23%) or epigastric pain (17%). These symptoms can be especially difficult to recognize immediately after the birth, especially if the woman has had an epidural. They can easily be ignored as being part of post-labour exhaustion.

Description of a seizure

Eclamptic seizures are described in different stages, though in reality these may all roll into one and be difficult to determine (Amiel 2012).

- Premonition: Suggested to be transient in nature and may be missed. The woman may roll her eyes, with facial and hand muscles twitching, and may cry out.
- Tonic stage: The woman's muscles go into spasm for about 30 seconds, with clenched fists and rigid arms and legs. The teeth are clenched and she may bite her tongue. Breathing will stop and her skin will become cyanosed.
- Clonic stage: Jerky, repetitive movements take place for about 2 minutes, with the body being thrown from side to side. Frothy, blood-stained saliva may come from the woman's mouth. Breathing is noisy and heavy, which may lead to inhalation of any mucous or blood present in her mouth.
- Coma: This may last from a few minutes to many hours, where the woman is deeply unconscious. Her face may remain swollen and congested although the cyanosis may fade.
- The onset may be very rapid, and immediate midwifery care is essential (see Table 7.1).

Medical treatment

Ideally, eclamptic seizures will have been prevented by previous recognition of severe pre-eclampsia and the preventative treatment with magnesium sulphate (Duley et al 2010a). However, as noted previously, some episodes of eclampsia may occur without any prior warning.

The management of eclampsia involves:

- Control of seizures
- Delivery of the infant, if not already accomplished
- Control of blood pressure
- Elimination of retained fluids
- Maintenance of adequate oxygen for the woman and baby (Amiel 2012)

Blood tests will be taken from the mother to establish a full picture of her condition, as severe pre-eclampsia and eclampsia have multisystem effects. An intravenous infusion will also be sited if not already in place. It is run slowly, initially, before administration of drugs.

Activity

Find out how a woman with known severe pre-eclampsia is cared for in your clinical area.

Establish what blood tests are usually taken in this situation and what equipment will be required.

Table 7.1: **Eclamptic seizures: immediate midwifery care**

Action	Rationale
Call for help.	Emergency situation: according to rules of practice.
Communicate with woman and partner about what is happening.	To try to keep her calm and alleviate stress – she will probably be able to hear what you are saying during the fit.
Place woman in left lateral position.	If antenatal, this reduces pressure of the uterus on the vena cava and allows continual bleed to flow to the fetus. If postnatal, this is the best possible position in which to keep her airway patent until assistance arrives.
Ensure any obstruction is removed from the mouth, gently using suction equipment if required.	To maintain a patent airway.
Aim to keep airway open.	To ensure as much oxygen is circulating as possible.
Give oxygen via a mask.	To ensure as much oxygen is circulating as possible for the mother and fetus.
Check vital signs – pulse and blood pressure.	Blood pressure may be causing the fit, or is it something else?
If antenatal, start/continue external/internal electronic monitoring.	To assess fetal well-being.
If postnatal ensure infant is safe with partner or other carer.	To ensure safety of the infant.
Explain what is happening and reassure any family members present.	To ensure psychological support for the woman and her family.
Insert urinary catheter and maintain hourly urinometer readings: aim to have an output of the previous hour + 30 ml.	To assess kidney function and monitor urine output.
Maintain strict fluid balance measurement.	To prevent dehydration or fluid overload.

Control of seizures

Management of eclamptic seizures reflects extensive research into the use of different drug regimes. The Collaborative Eclampsia Trial from 1991 to 1992 (Eclampsia Trial Collaborative Group 1995) carried out an international, multicentre trial which investigated the use of magnesium sulphate as an anticonvulsant versus either phenytoin or diazepam. The trial showed that magnesium sulphate reduced the number of seizures, with better outcomes for both mother and baby. More recent meta-analysis of trials shows that, in comparison with phenytoin and diazepam, magnesium sulphate is a more effective treatment and saves more lives from eclampsia (Duley et al 2010a, 2010b, 2010c).

Activity

Find out which intravenous solution is usually administered in your clinical area.

The recommended route of administration for magnesium sulphate is intravenously. The initial loading dose is 4 grams administered over 5 to 10 minutes followed by an infusion of 1 g/hour maintained for 24 hours (National Institute for Health and Care Excellence (NICE) 2010, 2011). If seizures continue a further dose of 2 to 4 grams may be given over 5 minutes.

Activity

It is recommended that every maternity unit should have prepared treatment packs available to manage this emergency. Locate where these are kept in your clinical area, what is kept in them and what the contents are used for.

During the administration of the drug, careful observation of the maternal respiration rate, urine output and patellar reflexes should be carried out because of the potential toxic effects of the drug which may lead to loss of reflexes and respiratory depression (Davey & Houghton 2013). Monitoring of blood serum levels of magnesium will also be required. Continuous monitoring of the fetal heart is also essential if the baby is not yet born (Davey & Houghton 2013). A further side effect may be flushing of the skin.

Control of blood pressure

The aim of reducing hypertension is to reduce the risk of cerebrovascular accident, strain on the heart and damage to the kidneys (Townsend et al

2016). The particular drug used will be related to the area of practice. NICE (2010, 2011) states that women with severe hypertension should be treated immediately with labetalol (oral or intravenous), hydralazine (intravenous) or nifedipine (oral).

Activity

Establish which drug is used to control hypertension in your area of practice.

What is the dosage and where is it kept?

The aim is to reduce the woman's systolic blood pressure to below 150 mm Hg and diastolic blood pressure to between 80 and 100 mm Hg and to maintain these levels (NICE 2010, 2011). Careful monitoring should take place to ensure the blood pressure falls and to assess if there are any adverse effects on the woman or her unborn baby, if in the antenatal period (NICE 2010, 2011). The fetal heart rate should be monitored continuously during the use of these drugs.

Activity

Check which equipment is required to provide care to women with complex medical needs.

Ensure you know how to use this correctly. How is it maintained and who is responsible for this?

Birth

If eclampsia occurs in the antenatal period, the aim will be to birth the infant once the mother's condition is stable. However, the midwife should also be aware of signs of imminent birth, especially if the seizures have taken place during labour. There should be a multidisciplinary approach to the care during the birth, including obstetricians, midwives, anaesthetists, neonatologists (especially if the infant is preterm) and intensive care specialist doctors. The decision regarding the safest method of birth will be determined depending on individual circumstances (NICE 2010, 2011). The midwife's role will include effective communication with the woman and her family to ensure that an appropriate explanation and psychological care are given.

Post-event

There should also be awareness of the increased risk of convulsions post-birth, and care will initially take place in a complicated care setting until the woman is in a stable condition. A midwife may be allocated to provide special care to the woman in the labour suite. Care of women with this condition should be in a quiet environment, and she should not be left alone during or after the event.

Monitoring for toxicity

Maternal observations should continue to be monitored and documented on a Modified Early Obstetric Warning System (MEOWS) chart. It is particularly important to continue to be vigilant for signs of magnesium toxicity, including:

+ Urine output < 20 ml/hour
+ Respiration rate < 14/minute
+ Oxygen saturation < 95%
+ Absent patella reflexes
+ Rising urea/creatinine

If toxicity is suspected then medical assistance should be sought. The infusion should be stopped and if mild toxicity, the woman's condition may right itself. If not, 10 ml of 10% calcium gluconate should be given intravenously SLOWLY over 10 minutes.

Observations

Accurate documentation of the event is essential and this should include: who was called, when they arrived, what actions were taken, along with all drugs given and maternal observations made. The observations need to be recorded regularly on a MEOWS chart, as well as in the woman's pregnancy record.

Care of the midwife who is looking after her should include support so that she receives adequate breaks, as it will be a stressful event for all involved. The multidisciplinary team may benefit from debriefing of the event and the care provided to ensure any learning may be achieved.

The woman may be transferred to an intensive care unit (ICU) if eclampsia occurs post-birth, and the midwife will liaise with the ICU staff to ensure that postnatal observations are continued and care is taken of the infant.

Care of the baby

If possible, an opportunity for the baby to be laid skin-to-skin with the woman should be taken before any transfer of the baby to a special care unit to promote well-being for both. Current advice for the use of hypertensive drugs and the relationship with lactation is dependent on the chosen drug (UK Drugs in Lactation Advisory Service 2017). Magnesium sulphate is thought to pass into breast milk but thought to be safe for the baby (Davey & Houghton 2013). Labetolol is also suggested to be safe (NICE

2010, 2011). Careful assessment will need to be made of the mother's condition to establish if it is appropriate to express and discard breast milk to stimulate lactation or for breastfeeding to occur.

Postnatal eclampsia

According to Douglas and Redman's (1994) population study there is a considerable risk of women developing eclampsia after 48 hours following birth. Postpartum eclampsia is less likely (Knight 2007), though it is still a possibility. It is therefore essential to observe closely women who have had signs of pre-eclampsia in the antenatal period. This is key in situations in which women are transferred home early into the community. Postnatal care plans should include information that enables women and families to recognize signs of raised blood pressure and to know whom to contact for support.

Further close liaison should be continued with general practitioners and obstetricians to ensure that women are reviewed and provided with appropriate ongoing medication and surveillance.

The midwife's role

Eclampsia is a serious condition, and it would be unusual in the UK for a midwife to care for women with this condition without medical support. Care will usually involve a team and multidisciplinary approach to care, with coordination by a senior doctor. However, the psychological care of the mother and her partner, and care of the infant, should be continued by the midwife, with awareness of the fear, anxiety and shock that the rapid onset of the condition may generate. The practical preparation of staff for the rare occurrence should be practised through drills locally to ensure competence if the need should arise (Ellis et al 2008). The use of multidisciplinary training for emergencies may improve the outcomes for infants (Draycott et al 2006) and can improve speed and efficiency (Thompson et al 2004). However, in relation to eclampsia, the rare and acute nature of the condition may mean that it is unnecessary to include all staff in the drills associated with its management (Thompson et al 2004).

> ### Activity
> What training is provided for staff in your locality in caring for women with this emergency?

What is clear is that midwives should be aware of their particular role in ensuring the safety, well-being and care of the woman, her infant and accompanying carers.

REFLECTION ON THE TRIGGER SCENARIO

Look back at the trigger scenario:

Keira gave birth to her first baby an hour and a half ago. She suddenly says, 'My eyes have gone blurred and I feel dizzy'. She collapses, and Val, the midwife caring for her, sees she has noticeable convulsive movements of her body.

Now that you are familiar with the principles of postpartum haemorrhage you should have some insight into the evidence and how the scenario relates to it. The jigsaw model will be used to explore the scenario in more depth.

Effective communication

Appropriate and effective communication is essential during times of emergency (NMC 2017). This will include communication with the woman and her family as well as appropriate referral to other members of the multi-professional team. Even though Keira is in a state of collapse she may still be able to hear, and it is important Val continues to communicate with her about what is happening. She also needs to communicate with the partner or those in the room to explain the circumstances. Val also needs to get help from the multidisciplinary team. Questions that could be asked are: Who will Val call for assistance and how will she communicate what has happened? How will she continue to communicate with Keira? How will she reassure her partner? Where and when will she record the event?

Using best evidence

In this circumstance it is important to be aware what the best evidence is surrounding the care of women during an eclamptic fit. Evidence has been presented in the preceding text of the best medical treatment to be used. Questions that could be asked are: Is this an eclamptic fit taking place or could it be something else? What is the best immediate care to be given by Val? What drugs are available in Val's working environment? Are there any further research trials being conducted into the care and treatment of women with hypertensive conditions in pregnancy? How do you keep up to date with new research findings?

Professional and legal issues

The midwife should always act professionally within her scope of practice (NMC 2017) and according to the law. Questions that could be asked are:

What is Emily's responsibility as a midwife regarding complex care situations? In what circumstances can care be given without Keira's consent? How will Val ensure she is acting within the Code of practice (NMC 2015). What is her duty of care regarding Keira's baby and her partner? What is the law regarding Keira's choices regarding her care? Can Keira refuse to have further treatment?

Team working

There will usually be a team of colleagues available for support within a hospital maternity unit. Midwives do not generally work in isolation but are part of a wider multidisciplinary team. Midwives working in the community will need to rely on the swift response of the emergency services in this situation, providing immediate transfer to the nearest maternity unit for obstetric care. Questions that could be asked are: In this circumstance, who are the members of the multidisciplinary team Val can call on? When should Val tell them and how? Who is responsible for Keira's ongoing care? What are Val's responsibilities in this team? Has the team undertaken multi-professional training for this situation?

Clinical dexterity

In this situation Val will need to employ her clinical dexterity to assess well-being and provide emergency treatment for this serious condition. She will need to make accurate assessments of Keira's condition and be able to support the administration of drug therapy. Questions that could be asked are: In this scenario what are Val's immediate clinical responsibilities? What observations should be carried out? How will she ensure that Keira's dignity and privacy are maintained? What emergency treatment may she commence? Has she had appropriate opportunities to practise emergency care of this kind?

Woman-centred care

It is expected that a woman should be central to the midwife's care. In this circumstance, it will be impossible to obtain consent and provide information in order for the woman to make choices about her care. However, it is essential to recognize the humanity of the woman and promote her well-being and dignity at all times, during and after the event. Questions that could be asked are: How can Val ensure that Keira is central to the actions she will take? How will Val promote Keira's dignity and well-being while emergency treatment is being carried out? How will the well-being of the mother–baby dyad be promoted? How will Keira's birth partner's emotional and information needs be catered for and by whom?

Models of care

The model of care that Keira has chosen may ultimately influence the nature of the response to an emergency situation. It is therefore important that when women choose where to have their baby, they are aware of the opportunities and restrictions that particular model presents. It is also key that women have had enough information about how emergency situations might be managed, in the unlikely event. Questions that may be asked are: Where did Keira birth her baby? Has Val been the midwife responsible for the birth? Who will be the lead professional for this circumstance? Who else is available in the room to help? If Keira birthed at home, how long will it take to transfer her to an obstetric unit? How will this transfer be facilitated?

Safe environment

When a birth is being planned, consideration should be made of the most appropriate environment for care of the individual woman and her baby. Whether this scenario was in a home, birth centre or hospital, a decision will need to be made regarding where Keira would be safest. In addition, with the current scenario, Keira and the baby need to be protected from further harm. Questions that may be asked are: Is Keira in the safest environment to protect her from harm? What will Val need to do to ensure Keira's safety during the seizure? Is the baby safe? What measures could Val have undertaken before the birth to prepare for this potential emergency event?

Promotes health

The aim of all maternity care is to promote the well-being of the woman and her baby. This will include her emotional, spiritual and social health as well as her physical needs. Questions that may be asked are: How will Keira's well-being as a new mother be promoted during this situation? How will Val help alleviate any anxieties she may have after the event or that of her partner? What steps can Val help Keira take to ensure her maximum health status in the future?

Who else might need to be involved in Keira's postnatal care to help her achieve this?

Further scenarios

Consider the following scenarios and think about how the specific situations may influence the care the midwife provides. Use the jigsaw model to explore the questions raised in each situation.

SCENARIO 1

Sharon is asking questions at the booking appointment of Ellen, who is pregnant with her first baby. She asks if there is anything Ellen knows about her family history that may be important. 'My mum said she had something called toxaemia when she had me'.

Practice point

When women offer information about their family history it is important to take notice, as it may be causing her some anxiety. The midwife should also be aware of relevant hereditary factors that may affect the woman and her potential care. In this scenario Sharon should be aware that 'toxaemia' refers to 'pre-eclamptic toxaemia', or PET, which is an older term for pre-eclampsia.

- What further questions may Sharon ask to establish what happened?
- How will she explain this condition to Ellen?
- How may she reassure Ellen about the condition?
- How will she follow up Ellen subsequently in pregnancy?
- What symptoms may she look for during the pregnancy?
- When should Ellen be encouraged to seek further advice?

SCENARIO 2

Faith is the coordinating midwife for the community maternity service. She receives a call from the partner of Imani, a Nigerian-born woman. Imani says that this is her fifth day since she had given birth to twins and she had a serious headache, photophobia, epigastric pain and a number of episodes of vomiting. Imani was wondering whether to call the GP.

Practice point

Eclampsia may develop in the postnatal period with no prior history of any symptoms. When a midwife is contacted with the news that a woman is unwell, it is important she takes appropriate action to ensure that she is assessed and cared for in the most appropriate place.

- What are the predisposing factors for eclampsia?
- What other questions will Faith ask to establish the cause of the illness?
- Should this be acted upon immediately?
- Where is the best place for Imani to be taken for assessment and how should she get there?
- When being assessed what tests will be required for Imani?
- What first-line treatment may be required?

Conclusion

Eclampsia is a serious condition that usually follows on from signs and symptoms of pre-eclampsia. The sequelae of not identifying or treating these symptoms may be potentially life-changing. It is vital that midwives are prepared for the incidence of eclampsia and know how to initiate care and treatment to reduce the incidence of further harm occurring in the woman and her baby.

Resources

Action on Pre-eclampsia e-learning course. Available at: https://action-on-pre-eclampsia.org.uk/E-learning/Elearning_Oct2014.pdf

NICE (2010, 2011) Hypertension in pregnancy: diagnosis and management. Available at: https://www.nice.org.uk/guidance/cg107/chapter/1-Guidance#medical-management-of-severe-hypertension-or-severe-pre-eclampsia-in-a-critical-care-setting

Pre-eclampsia RCOG patient guidance. Available at: https://www.rcog.org.uk/globalassets/documents/patients/patient-information-leaflets/pregnancy/pi-pre-eclampsia.pdf

References

Amiel, G.J., 2012. Essential Obstetric Practice. Springer, London.

Bellizzi, S., Sobel, H.L., Ali, M.M., 2017. Signs of eclampsia during singleton deliveries and early neonatal mortality in low- and middle-income countries from three WHO regions. Int. J. Gynecol. Obstet. 139, 50–54.

Bothamley, J., Boyle, M., 2017. Hypertensive and medical disorders in pregnancy. In: MacDonald, S., Johnson, G. (Eds.), Mayes' Midwifery: A Textbook for Midwives, fifth ed. Elsevier, Oxford.

Davey, L., Houghton, D., 2013. The Midwife's Pocket Formulary. Churchill Livingstone, Edinburgh.

Douglas, K.A., Redman, C.W., 1994. Eclampsia in the United Kingdom. BMJ 309, 1395–1400.

Draycott, T., Sibanda, T., Owen, L., et al., 2006. Does training in obstetric emergencies improve neonatal outcome? BJOG 113, 177–182.

Duley, L., Henderson-Smart, D.J., Walker, G.J.A., Chou, D., 2010a. Magnesium sulphate versus diazepam for eclampsia. Cochrane Database Syst. Rev. (12), CD000127, doi:10.1002/14651858.CD000127.pub2.CO000127.

Duley, L., Henderson-Smart, D.J., Chou, D., 2010b. Magnesium sulphate versus phenytoin for eclampsia. Cochrane Database Syst. Rev. (10), CD000128, doi:10.1002/14651858.CD000128.pub2.

Duley, L., Gülmezoglu, A.M., Chou, D., 2010c. Magnesium sulphate versus lytic cocktail for eclampsia. Cochrane Database Syst. Rev. (9), CD002960.

Eclampsia Trial Collaborative Group, 1995. Which anticonvulsant for women with eclampsia? Evidence from the Collaborative Eclampsia Trial. Lancet 345, 1455–1463.

Ellis, D., Crofts, J.F., Hunt, L.P., et al., 2008. Hospital, simulation center, and teamwork training for eclampsia management: a randomized controlled trial. Obstet. Gynecol. 111, 723–731.

Knight, M., 2007. Eclampsia in the United Kingdom 2005. BJOG 114, 1072–1078.

Knight, M., Nair, M., Tuffnell, D., et al. on behalf of MBRRACE-UK. Saving Lives, Improving Mothers' Care (Eds.), 2016. Surveillance of maternal deaths in the UK 2012-14 and lessons learned to inform maternity care from the UK and Ireland Confidential Enquiries into Maternal Deaths and Morbidity 2009–14. National Perinatal Epidemiology Unit, University of Oxford, Oxford.

Magpie Trial Collaborative Group, 2002. Do women with pre-eclampsia, and their babies, benefit from magnesium sulphate? The Magpie Trial: a randomised placebo-controlled trial. Lancet 359, 1877–1890.

National Institute for Health and Care Excellence (NICE), 2010, 2011. Hypertension in pregnancy: diagnosis and management. Available at: https://www.nice.org.uk/guidance/cg107/chapter/1-Guidance#medical-management-of-severe-hypertension-or-severe-pre-eclampsia-in-a-critical-care-setting.

Nursing and Midwifery Council (NMC), 2015. The Code for Nurses and Midwives. Nursing and Midwifery Council, London.

Nursing and Midwifery Council (NMC), 2017. Standards for competence for registered midwives. Avaiable at: https://www.nmc.org.uk/globalassets/sitedocuments/standards/nmc-standards-for-competence-for-registered-midwives.pdf.

Poon, L.C., Nicolaides, K.H., 2014. Early prediction of preeclampsia. Obstet. Gynecol. Int. 2014, 297397.

Roberts, C.L., Ford, J.B., Algert, C.S., et al., 2011. Population-based trends in pregnancy hypertension and pre-eclampsia: an international comparative study. BMJ Open 1, e000101.

Say, L., Chou, D., Gemmill, A., et al., 2014. Global causes of maternal death: a WHO systematic analysis. Lancet Global Health 2, e323–e333.

Shenone, M., Miller, D., Samson, J., et al., 2013. Eclampsia characteristics and outcomes: a comparison of two eras. J Pregnancy Available at: http://dx.doi.org/10.1155/2013/826045.

Steegers, E.A.P., von Dadelszen, P., Duvekot, J.J., Pijnenborg, R., 2010. Pre-eclampsia. Lancet 376, 631–644.

Subramaniam, V., 2007. Seasonal variation in the incidence of preeclampsia and eclampsia in tropical climatic conditions. BMC Womens Health 7, 18.

Thompson, S., Neal, S., Clark, V., 2004. Clinical risk management in obstetrics: eclampsia drills. BMJ 328, 269–271.

Townsend, R., O'Brien, P., Khalil, A., 2016. Current best practice in the management of hypertensive disorders in pregnancy. Integrat Blood Pressure Control 9, 79–94.

UK Drugs in Lactation Advisory Service. 2017. General principles for medicine use during breastfeeding. Available at: https://www.sps.nhs.uk/articles/ukdilas-general-principles-for-medicine-use-during-breastfeeding/.

Zeeman, G.G.1., Hatab, M.R., Twickler, D.M., 2004. Increased cerebral blood flow in preeclampsia with magnetic resonance imaging. Am. J. Obstet. Gynecol. 191, 1425–1429.

CHAPTER 8

Psychiatric emergencies

TRIGGER SCENARIO

Sarah, a community midwife, receives a telephone call from Simon. His partner, Wendy, gave birth to her first baby five days previously. 'I am really worried about her,' he says. 'She hasn't been sleeping well for days and now, today, she is forgetting to care for the baby and saying really odd things. She keeps talking really quickly and can't seem to sit still.'

Introduction

This book so far has explored some of the physical emergencies that midwives might encounter. This chapter describes the complex phenomenon of psychiatric emergency that may affect some childbearing women. The issues discussed here are rare; however, the recognition and prompt response to the signs of psychiatric illness are essential to the well-being of the mother and her baby. (Alongside this chapter the reader could also refer to Chapter 6, "Monitoring women's emotional well-being in the antenatal period" in Volume 2: Antenatal care and Chapter 8, "Emotional well-being following birth" in Volume 4: Postnatal care.)

Impaired mental health

Impaired mental health in pregnancy and after childbirth can range from being a mild, transient condition to a severe psychiatric emergency (Baston & Hall 2017). A serious mental illness (SMI) emergency has sudden onset with behaviours or emotional responses that may be life-threatening (Essali et al 2013). It may occur in women who have had previous, known psychiatric conditions, but also may occur suddenly for the first time after pregnancy. The pre-existing impaired mental health may have had an insidious onset after a prolonged period of less severe forms of illness. During pregnancy those women with pre-existing conditions may become less unwell during pregnancy, with less need for psychiatric referral, whereas women who develop conditions later in pregnancy are more likely to become more seriously ill (Raynor & Oates 2014).

In this area how many cases of puerperal psychosis might there be each year?

Women with pre-existing mental illness, and their families, will often have contact with other members of the multidisciplinary team, and the midwife will become one member of that team. For conditions that develop rapidly after childbirth, other professionals will be unlikely to be involved initially and the midwife may be the first health professional who observes changes in the woman's condition. These conditions may be a severe form of depressive illness or puerperal psychosis (Raynor & Oates 2014). Depression has been explored previously (Baston & Hall 2017); this chapter will focus in more depth on the psychotic condition that is thought to relate specifically to childbirth.

Postnatal or puerperal psychosis

This condition is an acute psychiatric emergency and is the most dramatic form of postnatal affective disorder (Raynor & England 2010). It is characterized by sudden onset. The timing of the onset is thought to be as early as 1 to 2 days after birth and within the first 2 weeks (Royal College of Psychiatrists (RCPsych) 2015). Oates (2004: 222) suggests that 80% will have an onset of 3 to 14 days, with day 5 being the most common, while Blackmore et al (2006) state that 97% had an onset within 2 weeks of the birth. The timing of the onset is significant, as women are often transferred home from postnatal wards within a day or two of the birth and community-based midwives may see the woman only 3 to 4 times before she is transferred to the care of the health visitor. The sudden nature of the condition may mean that women and their partners should be provided with information in order to recognize if any unusual psychological changes take place. National Institute for Health and Care Excellence (NICE) antenatal guidance (2008, 2017) advises discussing potential mental well-being disorders at the 36-week appointment during pregnancy.

Discover what information about mental well-being is given to women and their partners at the 36-week antenatal appointment and after the birth.

Find out the usual pattern of postnatal care provided by community midwives locally.

As indicated previously, the condition is rare, affecting one or two women per 1000 births (RCPsych 2015). However, this may be in specific populations of women whose illness requires them to be admitted to hospital. In the whole population there could be more who do not go for treatment. The risk for a woman's first experience of psychosis is thought to be 23 times higher in the first 4 weeks postnatal compared with any other period during a woman's life (Bergink et al 2016). The risk of postpartum psychosis increases considerably if the woman has had a psychotic episode in the antenatal period (Harlow et al 2007) or if there is a history of psychosis in her family (Cantwell et al 2017).

The seriousness of mental disturbance after childbirth is highlighted by Confidential Enquiries into Maternal Death in the UK (Knight et al 2017), which have demonstrated that women with mental illness are at high risk of committing suicide after giving birth. Furthermore, the infant and other children of women with disturbed mental well-being may be at high risk of rejection or abuse (Brockington 2004), with some situations leading to infanticide (Brockington 2017).

Risk factors

Women during their first pregnancy are thought to be most at risk (Bergink et al 2016). Of the women who developed puerperal psychosis in the study of Blackmore et al (2006), 82% were primiparous. It has also been suggested that sleep deprivation can precipitate manic mood states, with the indication that for susceptible first-time mothers after long labours this may be a risk factor (Sharma et al 2004). There is also evidence that some women susceptible to bipolar illness may experience psychotic episodes after menstruation or termination of pregnancy (Brockington 2004). The aetiology of this is not clear, with suggestions of a relationship with immunological responses, or hormonal or biological reasons (Blackmore et al 2006).

There appears to be a genetic and familial factor to the condition, with women at risk who have had a personal history of affective psychosis, a previous history of puerperal psychosis or a close relation with affective psychosis (Cantwell & Cox 2003; Brockington 2004). However, there are complex factors that underpin the development of the condition (Bergink et al 2016; Inglis et al 2017). Social and life events do not appear to be linked to risk of development of psychosis (Bergink et al 2016), though there does appear to be some connection with preterm birth and caesarean section (Nager et al 2008).

In a study of Swedish women, hospitalization for serious psychiatric conditions was associated with higher age groups and with not living with the father of the child (Nager et al 2005). The authors suggest that the former may be related to hormonal or biological factors, and that this is

Table 8.1: **Symptoms of psychosis**

Depressive	Manic	Psychotic
Frequent tearfulness	Overactivity	Delusions
Sadness	Elated	Visual or auditory
Suicidal ideas	Over-talkative	Hallucinations
Poor appetite	Restlessness	Intrusive thoughts
Poor sleep	Irritability	Unusual beliefs
Poor concentration	Disorientation in time, place, person	Non-recognition and non-identification of those around

significant with the current rising age group of first-time mothers in developed populations. Furthermore, they indicate that single women will have less social support and increased sleep deprivation.

Symptoms and clinical picture

Postnatal psychotic conditions are manifest by women appearing well initially, but who may then become extremely depressed or psychotic very quickly (Bergink et al 2016). Potential signs and symptoms of the condition are presented in Table 8.1.

The bizarre and erratic nature of the symptoms may alert family members or health carers that the woman is acting strangely and requires help. However, care should be taken to establish as full a history as possible because other psychiatric disorders may manifest with psychotic-like symptoms. Also, medical conditions such as thyroiditis, sepsis or the use of addictive drugs such as ecstasy or LSD may act as triggers to symptoms that appear psychiatric in origin (Miller 2002).

Preventative measures

Antenatal care

Midwives are in a strong position to recognize any changes in the mental well-being of the mother, but the role of the midwife in preventing mental illness in childbearing women should not be underestimated. Creating a service where women and their families are supported effectively will enable women to feel empowered, promote positive emotional health (Baston & Hall 2017) and allow changes from normal patterns to be observed, with rapid referral to further agencies as required.

Careful questioning at the initial booking will ensure identification of those women most at risk of postnatal mental illness. Those women with current illness, known previous psychosis or strong family history should be specifically identified (Scottish Intercollegiate Guidelines Network (SIGN) 2012; Cantwell et al 2017). They will require early referral to psychiatric services and will be cared for within a multidisciplinary framework. A multidisciplinary individualized plan of care should be created, with a copy kept in her handheld records.

The aim of care will be to maintain support in the community, so the family practitioner will be involved as well as, potentially, community psychiatric nurses: there will also be early involvement of health visitors and, potentially, social workers. Liaison between these team members should be frequent; however, the midwife should maintain high-quality midwifery care and support. The woman's and her family's knowledge of her condition should not be underestimated, and she should be included in all aspects of communication regarding the decisions about her pregnancy and after the birth. Families should be included in discussions to ensure the woman has appropriate social support and that they have clear understanding and lines of referral in case of deterioration (NICE 2014, 2017).

In women who are known to be particularly at risk, the provision of one-to-one care as much as possible in the antenatal period and through to the puerperium will mean that women and their families and midwives can build up effective relationships and mutual trust. This will lead to women feeling more safe and secure, with a subsequent reduction in anxiety and fear. However, during the provision of antenatal services it may be difficult to ensure continuity of carer throughout a pregnancy. It is therefore imperative that midwives maintain meticulous records and provide verbal handover to team members to ensure that women at risk are closely monitored and any deterioration in their health is swiftly identified.

A postnatal care plan should be established to ensure that strategies for swift referral and support are instigated. As a preventative measure, future practice may be to start prophylactic medication of women in high-risk groups during pregnancy, but the evidence base for this is currently insufficient (SIGN 2012).

Activity

Find out what provision of antenatal care is available for women with known mental health conditions in your locality. What are the referral criteria, and how soon can a mental health assessment be made?

Postnatal care

For all women in the postnatal period, sleep deprivation and fatigue may be factors in emotional well-being (Baston & Hall 2017). Sharma (2003) has suggested that sleep deprivation may be a factor in psychotic conditions. As preventative measures, she has suggested:

- Carefully observe the sleep–wake cycle of women with personal and family history of affective disorders during pregnancy and in the postnatal period.
- Aim to improve sleep through having a daytime birth.
- Have the newborn sleep in the nursery.
- Ensure early identification and treatment of insomnia in high-risk women.

The suggestion to induce labour to ensure birth happens in daylight hours may not be the most appropriate action if we consider the positive effects on women's well-being of a normal birth and on the relationship with the baby. Therefore appropriate discussion should take place with the obstetricians and psychiatric team to ensure the most appropriate care for the woman concerned. It is also debatable whether separation of the mother and baby in the postnatal period is the most appropriate course of action. Further study to ensure the best care needs to be carried out.

Wray (2011) identified that postnatal wards are not the best places for sleeping. However, there are ways that the potential for a restful environment can be maximized (Baston & Hall 2017):

- Recognition that sleep and rest are part of healing and restoration and vital to mental well-being
- Adapting 'routine' midwifery care to fit in with opportunity for sleep
- Taking steps to lower noise levels on wards at all times, especially at night, which could include the type of shoes midwives choose to wear, and lowering the volume of conversations, televisions and radios
- Repair of squeaking equipment
- Reduction of light levels at night
- Provision of written information to partners of the need for postnatal rest, which can also be passed on to other relatives

Early transfer home may also be beneficial, but continued careful observation by community staff should be ensured.

Care and treatment

In the acute phase of the condition, the focus of immediate care of the mother and the baby will be to ensure their safety. The woman should not be left alone at any time, and referral to perinatal mental health services is essential. In some cases, if the condition is first diagnosed on a postnatal ward the woman will be given initial treatment there while a psychiatric bed is located. The specialist perinatal health team should continue to monitor her condition and support the delivery of her care.

When a woman needs to be hospitalized to protect her safety, this can be achieved in a number of ways. She may need to be 'sectioned' for a period of time under the Mental Health Act (Great Britain 1983, updated 2007). The Mental Health Act makes various provisions for a range of circumstances, and these are each described and precisely defined in various 'sections' of the Act. Hence the term 'sectioned' is often used when a woman has been detained for her own safety or that of others.

Although navigating the Mental Health Act is complex, the most relevant sections are:

+ Section 1 provides definitions of mental disorders.
+ Section 2 refers to admission for assessment.
+ Section 3 refers to admission for treatment.

Activity

In what circumstances might a woman be sectioned under the Mental Health Act?

Who needs to be involved to make an application to detain under the Mental Health Act?

A woman may volunteer for assessment and treatment in a psychiatric facility. If she refuses such assessment, and is deemed to be a danger to herself or others, she may be required to be detained under Section 2 of the Mental Health Act for Assessment. If following such assessment, she is deemed to require treatment (for example, with drugs or electroconvulsive therapy (ECT)) she can be detained under Section 3 of the Act for this care.

If a woman lacks capacity to consent, the powers of the Mental Health Act are not required to provide physical care and treatment, as this can be sanctioned in her best interest, under the Mental Capacity Act (2005). However, if treatment is required for her mental ill health, the Mental Health Act is used (RCPsych 2014). If her physical health condition is contributing to or is a result of her mental illness, her physical illness can also be treated under the Mental Health Act (Jones 2017). See Table 8.2 for a summary of when the mental health acts can be used.

Activity

Consider the potential circumstances when a woman might be treated under the Mental Health Act for a physical illness that is detrimental to her mental health status.

Table 8.2: **Powers of the mental capacity and mental health acts**

Mental Capacity Act (2005)	Mental Health Act (1983, 2007)
Physical or mental illness leading to lack of capacity such that a person is: • Unable to make decisions for themselves about care and treatment • Making decisions they would not make if they were well	Mental illness such that a person is: • A risk to themselves or others, or seriously unwell • Declining treatment, but could still have capacity
Powers: Doctors and nurses can give a physical treatment against a person's will in their best interest.	**Powers:** Psychiatrist can treat mental illness against a person's will, having applied for such under the Mental Health Act.

Mother and baby units

The gold standard is that the woman and her baby will be hospitalized together in a special mother and baby unit (MBU) and cared for by a team of specialist practitioners. The ultimate aim is to keep the mother and baby united, although there are a limited number of psychiatric units that provide such facilities and admission to a general psychiatric ward may be the only alternative. If this is the case, care by close relatives or foster care will need to be arranged for the baby.

There are just 15 MBUs for the whole of England; hence there are plans to expand existing provision and create further new facilities (NHS England 2017). In addition, there is a pledge that 'by 2020/21, NHSE will support 30,000 more woman each year to access evidence-based specialist mental health care during the perinatal period' (Mental Health Taskforce 2016: 33).

For most women, there is evidence that parenting and clinical outcomes are good after treatment in MBUs, with the exception of those women with schizophrenic conditions (Gillham & Wittkowski 2015). According to NICE (2014, 2017) specialist perinatal inpatient services should:

+ Provide facilities designed specifically for mothers and babies (typically with 6–12 beds)
+ Be staffed by specialist perinatal mental health staff
+ Be staffed to provide appropriate care for babies
+ Have effective liaison with general medical and mental health services
+ Have available the full range of therapeutic services
+ Be closely integrated with community–based mental health services to ensure continuity of care and minimum length of stay.

It should be ensured that the MBU is the most appropriate place. If the woman is acutely ill, she may pose a risk to herself, her baby and to other mothers and babies in the unit. She may therefore need to be cared for in a more secure setting temporarily until she is more stable.

> ### Activity
> Find out about the nearest MBU in your area. How many beds does it have, and how wide a geographical area does it serve?

A midwife's role in relation to the emergency will involve support of the family during admission and continuing to provide postnatal care in the hospital.

Therapies

The aim of care will involve restoration of the woman's self-confidence, enabling her to build a relationship with the infant and develop mothering skills. The types of medication will include a combination of drugs from the antidepressant, mood stabilizing or neuroleptic groups of drugs (SIGN 2012). The use of drugs will have an effect on the woman's ability to breastfeed and therefore the choice of treatment will take this into consideration (NICE 2014, 2017).

In some cases, ECT may also be used in situations in which her health or that of her unborn baby is at serious risk (NICE 2014, 2017).

> ### Activity
> Find out about ECT and how this is thought to work. Where is this therapy administered? What does the procedure involve?

As the woman begins to recover, talking therapies based on a cognitive-behavioural therapy (CBT) model may be useful to help her modify the way she behaves in response to unhelpful thoughts.

Social support

After a psychotic event, time and care should be given to the partner and family members who will be shocked by the experience. Women appear to recover better if they have good social support (McGrath et al 2013); therefore opportunities to discuss the event and the future progress of the symptoms will need to be explored. There is evidence that relationships are severely strained by the condition, which occurs at a vulnerable time (Robertson & Lyons 2003), and explanation and support may go some way to assist in maintaining relationships. Also, staff and students who have been involved should be supported effectively, as this may be a rare and traumatic occurrence (Price 2004). Safeguarding procedures may also need to be instigated for the protection of the infant and any other children, as there is potential of harm to them or to the woman herself (SIGN 2012).

> **Activity**
>
> Find out about the local support groups that exist for women affected by severe mental illness. Where do they meet and how often?

Women's experiences

Although postnatal depression has been highly researched, psychotic conditions have received less attention. Knowledge of women's experiences of the condition is also limited. A qualitative study (Robertson & Lyons 2003) examined women's experiences of puerperal psychosis, aiming to 'gain understanding into living through and past the illness'. The researchers interviewed 10 women with onset of the illness within 6 weeks of birth in the previous 10 years. The women thus had a long-term view of the condition. Three of the women had given birth to another child since the experience, and had been unaffected by a further psychotic episode. The women in this study identified that the illness was different and 'separate' from other forms of mental illness, where they required:

+ Specialized treatment to identify with others going through the experience to 'normalize' what was happening to them

They felt isolated and afraid. There was also identification of loss of:

+ Control over decisions, treatment and themselves
+ Motherhood
+ The mother and child relationship
+ Further pregnancies and children

Relationships also suffered, with the partner relationship deteriorating and the mother needing to choose between the baby and the partner. Furthermore, other members of the family and friends experienced distress and reacted negatively towards them. The researchers established that these women had to learn to live with their emotions and to regain their sense of self after the illness. They conclude that further research needs to be carried out which would include exploring the views and experiences of partners and family members, as the illness affects all relationships within the woman's life (Robertson & Lyons 2003).

A further qualitative study with 12 women identified the different processes for recovery from the experience that included developing understanding and coming to terms with what had happened to them (McGrath et al 2013). Women and their families need information regarding the long-term effect of the condition, as further hospital admissions might be appropriate (Garfield et a1 2004), with the ability to recognize when additional help might be required.

REFLECTION ON THE TRIGGER SCENARIO

Look back at the trigger scenario:

> Sarah, a community midwife, receives a telephone call from Simon. His partner, Wendy, gave birth to her first baby five days previously. 'I am really worried about her,' he says. 'She hasn't been sleeping well for days and now, today, she is forgetting to care for the baby and saying really odd things. She keeps talking really quickly and can't seem to sit still.'

Now that you are familiar with a psychiatric emergency you should have some insight into the evidence and how the scenario relates to it. The jigsaw model will be used to explore the scenario in more depth.

Effective communication

When caring for any women it is important to use appropriate communication skills, especially so when assessing for or dealing with an emergency situation. Effective communication is vital in relation to mental well-being and receiving information from family members. In this circumstance, the midwife is receiving information via a telephone. Questions that may be considered in this scenario are: Has Sarah already developed a relationship with Simon and Wendy? What questions should Sarah ask about Wendy? Can Sarah speak to Wendy on the telephone? What questions could she ask her to establish her well-being? What clues could be obtained from what and how Wendy replies? How should Sarah record the discussion? Should Sarah visit Wendy, and if so, when?

Woman-centred care

Ensuring sensitive, individualized care for women is essential for all women, including those with serious mental wellbeing concerns. It is vital in order to recognize when increased support is required from the midwife or from the multidisciplinary team to the woman and to the wider family. In this scenario what could be asked are: Have there been any concerns raised about Wendy before by Simon or other professionals? Has she been included in plans about her care and asked what her needs are? Has Sarah met Wendy before and built up a relationship? How will Sarah ensure Wendy is included in decisions about her care?

Using best evidence

In this scenario, the midwife needs to use the best evidence available to make decisions about appropriate care for Wendy. Questions that need to be addressed to ensure that the woman's care is evidence based include: What questions will Sarah ask to establish what is happening to Wendy? How will she identify the condition? What is the evidence around the causes of postnatal psychosis? What evidence is there about appropriate forms of care or treatment? How will Sarah use National Guidelines to provide the most appropriate care for Wendy?

Professional and legal

Midwives should always practice within professional frameworks and the law. In this scenario questions that need to be addressed to ensure that the woman's care fulfils statutory obligations include: Has Sarah undertaken appropriate training in relation to mental health assessment and to recognize psychosis? How do the standards of practice and code of professional conduct help her in providing care for Wendy? Are there any national or international guidelines appropriate to Wendy's care? What are Deprivation Of Liberty Safeguards (DOLS)?

Team working

Community-based midwives do not work in isolation, although they must exercise individual professional responsibility for their actions. They are usually based in a primary health environment and have connections with and to other health professionals. Questions that need to be addressed in this scenario are: Are Wendy and Simon's needs significant to warrant inviting involvement of other professionals? If so, who will this be? How will Sarah make contact with them and when? Where will information be recorded for other health professionals? Who will be the lead professional caring for Wendy?

Clinical dexterity

In relation to complex emotional issues, clinical skills usually may not be required; however, if the midwife needs to carry out any tests following on from the discussion she should use sensitivity and gentleness. Questions that could arise: Could there be a clinical basis for Wendy's behaviour? Does Sarah need to make any clinical assessments in relation to Wendy's care? If so, what might those include? What are the normal ranges for these assessments? Where should these clinical assessments be undertaken? Should she carry out any clinical examination of the baby?

Models of care

In relation to postnatal care there are currently a number of models that midwives work with in the UK. Ideally complex emotional or psychiatric needs are best cared for by carers known to the woman and her family. How care is organized may have a positive or negative effect on the emotional well-being of some women. In this scenario, questions that could be raised are: Does Sarah work in a team of colleagues who aim to provide continuity through the whole pregnancy continuum? Has she developed a relationship with Simon and Wendy during the pregnancy and therefore is the appropriate midwife to care for her? Would continuity be beneficial in this situation? Is home-based care more beneficial in this situation or should she receive in-hospital care? Are there other professional groups already involved in the provision of the care Sarah is giving?

Safe environment

Midwifery care should be carried out in the safest environment, for the woman, her baby, family members and also for the midwife. The unpredictable nature of certain mental health conditions means that midwives should be vigilant to ensure safety is maintained. Questions that could be asked about this scenario are: Are Wendy and her baby currently in a safe environment in her home or are there reasons to believe she may be putting herself or her family at risk? Would Sarah be safe to visit Wendy at home as a lone professional or should she attend with someone else? Where could a safe environment be for Wendy and her baby?

Promotes health

All midwifery care should provide the opportunity to promote the holistic health of a woman, her family and the community in which they work. In this scenario questions that could be asked to ensure that the woman's care promotes health include: Are there circumstances that have triggered Wendy's current behaviours apart from the birth of her baby? Does the environment where Wendy is living promote her mental well-being and that of Simon and their baby? Have her sleep and diet been adequate? Are there ways Sarah could promote Wendy's and Simon's emotional health at this time?

Further scenarios

SCENARIO 1

Maria has arrived for booking for her second pregnancy. In the previous maternity notes Emilia reads that Maria was admitted to a mother and baby unit 2 days after the birth of her previous baby and stayed there for 5 months.

Practice point

After a prior experience of a psychotic episode in a previous pregnancy the chance of a recurrence is high. In this circumstance, the midwife should be vigilant to the history and be prepared to discuss this with Maria and her family.

What questions will Emilia ask and how will she ask them?

+ Has she already met Maria in previous pregnancy?
+ If not, has Maria built up a relationship with a different midwife who could be her primary carer?
+ Is Maria experiencing any fear relating to this previous experience, and how may Emilia support her through this?
+ What model of care is best in this circumstance over her pregnancy?
+ Who should Maria be referred to with her permission?
+ What is the midwife's responsibility in the multidisciplinary team?
+ How will information be recorded in the booking notes?

SCENARIO 2

Andy is a midwife working on the postnatal ward. He hears a baby crying continuously. On walking behind a curtain in a four-bed room he discovers the baby lying exposed without a nappy in the cot and April, her mother, lying on the bed with her back to the baby. When he walks round to see her face he notes she is staring ahead blankly, apparently oblivious to the noise of the baby.

Practice point

Serious psychological reactions in the postnatal period may happen within 24 hours of birth and therefore could occur on the postnatal ward. The effect on the mother may be such that she is unaware of the needs of her baby. Safety of the woman and baby, and well-being of the other women within the ward area should be paramount.

Questions that could be asked in this circumstance are:

+ How will Andy establish what the needs of April and her baby are at this time?
+ How may her condition be diagnosed?

- What has triggered this reaction for her?
- What type of birth did she have and does she need physical care that is affecting her?
- Which members of the multidisciplinary team will Andy discuss April's care with?
- Where is the safest environment for April's continuing care?
- How will April's family be involved in her care?

Conclusion

Postnatal psychotic illness is a serious condition that may take everyone by surprise. This chapter has highlighted that midwives should be alert in their care of women who have a strong family history of mental disturbance related to childbirth or who have known long-term mental health difficulties. Further services should be in place to ensure that postnatal support is available for all women and their families. Provision of appropriate information about who to contact if families are concerned will ensure that women receive rapid treatment on the rare occasion that their mental health seriously deteriorates.

Resources
Action on postpartum psychosis
https://www.app-network.org/
Association for Postnatal Illness
https://apni.org/
The International Marce Society for Perinatal Health
https://marcesociety.com/
MIND
https://www.mind.org.uk/
Postnatal illness
http://www.pni.org.uk/
BBC tv programme My baby, psychosis and me
http://www.bbc.co.uk/programmes/b07187xv
Perinatal mental health toolkit
http://www.rcgp.org.uk/clinical-and-research/toolkits/perinatal-mental-health-toolkit.aspx
Management of perinatal mood disorders
http://www.sign.ac.uk/sign-127-management-of-perinatal-mood-disorders.html

References
Baston, H., Hall, J., 2017. Midwifery Essentials, vol. 4. Postnatal Care. Elsevier, Oxford.

Bergink, V., Rasgon, N., Wisner, K.L., 2016. Postpartum psychosis: madness, mania, and melancholia in motherhood. Am. J. Psychiatry 173, 1179–1188.

Blackmore, E.R., Jones, I., Doshi, M., et al., 2006. Obstetric variables associated with bipolar affective puerperal psychosis. Br. J. Psychiatry 188, 32–36.

Brockington, I., 2004. Postpartum psychiatric disorders. Lancet 363, 303–310.

Brockington, I., 2017. Suicide and filicide in postpartum psychosis. Arch Womens Mental Health 20, 63–69.

Cantwell, R., Cox, J.L., 2003. Psychiatric disorders in pregnancy and puerperium. Curr Obstet Gynecol 13, 7–13.

Cantwell, R., Gray, R., Knight, M., on behalf of the MBRRACE-UK psychosis chapter-writing group. 2017. Caring for women with psychosis. In: Knight M, Nair M, Tuffnell D, et al, eds., Saving lives, improving mothers' care: lessons learned to inform maternity care from the UK and Ireland Confidential Enquiries into Maternal Deaths and Morbidity 2013–15. Available at: https://www.npeu.ox.ac.uk/downloads/files/mbrrace-uk/reports/MBRRACE-UK%20Maternal%20Report%202017%20-%20Web.pdf.

Essali, A., Alabed, S., Guul, A., Essali, N., 2013. Preventive interventions for postnatal psychosis. Cochrane Database Syst. Rev. (6), CD009991, doi:10.1002/14651858.CD009991.pub2.

Garfield, P., Kent, A., Paykel, E.S., et al., 2004. Outcome of postpartum disorders: a 10 year follow-up of hospital admissions. Acta Psychiatr. Scand. 109, 434–439.

Gillham, R., Wittkowski, A., 2015. Outcomes for women admitted to a mother and baby unit: a systematic review. Int J Womens Health 7, 459–476.

Great Britain, 1983. updated 2007. Mental Health Act. Her Majesty's Stationery Office, London.

Harlow, B.L., Vitonis, A.F., Sparen, P., et al., 2007. Incidence of hospitalization for postpartum psychotic and bipolar episodes in women with and without prior prepregnancy or prenatal psychiatric hospitalizations. Arch. Gen. Psychiatry 64, 42–48.

Inglis, A., Morris, E., Austin, J., 2017. Prenatal genetic counseling for psychiatric disorders. Prenat. Diagn. 37, 6–13.

Jones, R., 2017. Mental Health Act Manual, 20th ed. Sweet & Maxwell, London.

Knight, M., Nair, M., Tuffnell, D., et al., eds. 2017. Saving lives, improving mothers' care: lessons learned to inform maternity care from the UK and Ireland Confidential Enquiries into Maternal Deaths and Morbidity 2013–15. Available at: https://www.npeu.ox.ac.uk/downloads/files/mbrrace-uk/reports/MBRRACE-UK%20Maternal%20Report%202017%20-%20Web.pdf.

McGrath, L., Peters, S., Wieck, A., Wittkowski, A., 2013. The process of recovery in women who experienced psychosis following childbirth. BMC Psychiatry 13, 341.

Mental Health Taskforce. 2016. The five year forward view for mental health. Available at: https://www.england.nhs.uk/wp-content/uploads/2016/02/Mental-Health-Taskforce-FYFV-final.pdf.

Miller, L., 2002. Postpartum depression. JAMA 287, 762–765.

Nager, A., Johansson, L.M., Sundquist, K., 2005. Are sociodemographic factors and year of delivery associated with hospital admission for postpartum psychosis? A study of 500 000 first- time mothers. Acta Psychiatric Scand 112, 47–53.

Nager, A., Sundquist, K., Ramírez-León, V., Johansson, L.M., 2008. Obstetric complications and postpartum psychosis: a follow-up study of 1.1 million first-time mothers between 1975 and 2003 in Sweden. Acta Psychiatr. Scand. 117, 12–19.

National Institute for Health and Care Excellence (NICE). 2008, 2017. Antenatal care for uncomplicated pregnancies clinical guideline. Available at: https://www.nice.org.uk/guidance/cg62.

National Institute for Health and Care Excellence (NICE). 2014, 2017. Antenatal and postnatal mental health: clinical management and service guidance. Available at: https://www.nice.org.uk/guidance/cg192/chapter/1-Recommendations#principles-of-care-in-pregnancy-and-the-postnatal-period-2.

NHS England. 2017. Next steps on the NHS five year forward view. Available at: https://www.england.nhs.uk/2017/03/nhs-acts-to-cut-inappropriate-out-of-area-placements-for-children-and-young-people-in-mental-health-crisis/.

Oates, M.R., 2004. Psychiatric disorders of childbirth. In: Symonds, E.M., Symonds, I.M. (Eds.), Essential Obstetrics and Gynaecology. Churchill Livingstone, Edinburgh.

Price, S., 2004. Midwifery care and mental health. Pract. Midwife 7, 12–14.

Raynor, M.D., England, C., 2010. Psychology for Midwives: Pregnancy, Childbirth and Puerperium. Open University Press, Maidenhead.

Raynor, M.D., Oates, M.R., 2014. Perinatal mental health. In: Marshall, J., Raynor, M. (Eds.), Myles' Textbook for Midwives, 16th ed. Churchill Livingstone, Oxford.

Robertson, E., Lyons, A., 2003. Living with puerperal psychosis: a qualitative review. Psychol. Psychother. 76, 411–431.

Royal College of Psychiatrists (RCPsych). 2014. Capacity and the Mental Capacity Act (MCA). Available at: http://www.rcpsych.ac.uk/healthadvice/problemsanddisorders/mentalcapacityandthelaw.aspx.

Royal College of Psychiatrists (RCPsych). 2015. Postpartum psychosis: severe mental illness after childbirth. Available at: http://www.rcpsych.ac.uk/healthadvice/problemsanddisorders/postpartumpsychosis.aspx.

Scottish Intercollegiate Guidelines Network (SIGN Executive). 2012. Management of perinatal mood disorders: a national clinical guideline. Available at: http://www.sign.ac.uk/assets/sign127.pdf.

Sharma, V., 2003. Role of sleep loss in the causation of puerperal psychosis. Med Hypoth 61, 477–481.

Sharma, V., Smith, A., Khan, M., 2004. The relationship between duration of labour, time of delivery, and puerperal psychosis. J. Affect. Disord. 83, 215–220.

Wray, J., 2011. Bouncing Back? An Ethnographic Study Exploring the Context of Care and Recovery After Birth Through the Experiences and Voices of Mothers. PhD thesis, University of Salford.

CHAPTER 9

Uterine emergencies

Ruptured uterus, scar dehiscence, inverted uterus

Alison Brodrick

TRIGGER SCENARIO

Chrissie is expecting her second child and is anxious about giving birth again, as her first child was born by caesarean section after a long labour. At the booking appointment she asks her community midwife if she will be OK this time and if she can try again for a homebirth. Her midwife tells her that there is a risk of scar rupture and that she must give birth in a hospital; she reassures her that an obstetrician will discuss it all with her at the hospital and if she wants she could just have a repeat caesarean. Afterwards the community midwife says to her student midwife, 'Once you have seen a rupture it makes you really cautious.'

Introduction

Uterine emergencies in obstetrics can be fatal. The most common uterine emergency is atony leading to postpartum haemorrhage, which is discussed in Chapter 6. Less common are a ruptured uterus, wound dehiscence and inverted uterus. Although rare, it is important that the student midwife can recognize and act appropriately. Uterine inversion is uncommon and not something that women tend to discuss. Uterine rupture, on the other hand, is more widely raised and can be an emotive topic for women considering birth after caesarean. It is important that the student midwife understands the evidence and can allay fears appropriately. This chapter will explore the risk factors, symptoms and management of these uterine emergencies.

Ruptured uterus

A complete rupture of the uterus is rare. It can occur at any time during labour and involves the full thickness of the uterine wall and pelvic peritoneum. It can be sudden and dramatic, with fetal parts escaping into the peritoneal cavity; it requires immediate action to save the lives of the mother and the baby. More common and less dramatic is an incomplete rupture, also referred to as dehiscence or a 'silent rupture'. This involves the myometrium but not the pelvic peritoneum. It also requires immediate action; however, as the term 'silent' suggests, women are often asymptomatic and it may not be discovered until much later. The term 'rupture' is often used interchangeably to mean both 'complete' and 'incomplete' and this needs to be noted when reviewing the evidence. The UK Obstetric Surveillance System (UKOSS) (Fitzpatrick et al 2012) reports the incidence of true complete rupture in the UK as 0.2 per 1000 of all deliveries. For women wishing to labour after a primary caesarean section the risk rises to 2.1 per 1000 or 1 in 500 (0.2%). In the MBRRACE UK 2009 to 2012 report, four women died as a result of uterine rupture, none had a scar on the uterus and three of the cases involved oxytocic use to augment or induce labour (Knight et al 2014).

Activity

Think about your own views and knowledge of uterine rupture. Does this affect how you convey information to women in the antenatal period? If so, how and why do you think this is?

Risk factors

In the developing world the main risk is an obstructed labour and limited access to obstetric care in labour (Oyston et al 2014).

In the developed world, although an obstructed labour does increase the risk of rupture, the main risk factor is a previous lower section caesarean section; if it is a classical incision the risk is higher. There remains some professional contention regarding vaginal birth after two or more caesareans. Current figures suggest the rate of rupture rises to 1.36% (Tahseen & Griffiths 2010), with an increased risk of hysterectomy and blood transfusion. It is therefore important that an individual assessment should be made which includes planned size of family, as the risk of repeat caesarean must also appreciate the additional risks of placenta accreta and placenta praevia in subsequent pregnancies.

Other risk factors include:

+ Scarring or perforation of the uterus from previous uterine surgery
+ Misuse of oxytocin and/or prostaglandins
+ Use of instruments
+ Intrauterine manipulations
+ Placental abruption due to distension of the uterine wall
+ Grand multiparity

Symptoms of complete uterine rupture can be very sudden and feature some or all of the following:

+ Maternal collapse
+ Fetal distress

- Fetus palpated in the abdomen
- Constant abdominal pain
- Contractions slow or stop

All of the foregoing symptoms can also apply to incomplete rupture (apart from the fetus being palpated in the abdomen). As already discussed, however, the symptoms of an incomplete rupture can be more difficult to recognize and may be diagnosed only after the birth. Additional symptoms can include:

- Scar tenderness
- Maternal tachycardia
- Vaginal bleeding
- Shoulder pain
- Anxiety
- Restlessness
- Dizziness

Although scar tenderness is often cited as a symptom of uterine rupture, it does not present in all cases. A more significant feature is a non-reassuring fetal heart rate tracing, typically with significant variable decelerations and/or bradycardia and present in 76% of cases reported in the UK Obstetric Surveillance System data (Fitzpatrick et al 2012). Using continuous fetal heart monitoring is therefore recommended for all women labouring with a previous caesarean scar.

Activity

Ask the midwives in your maternity unit if they have seen a true 'rupture' and explore professionals' attitudes towards vaginal birth after caesarean (VBAC). Are they familiar with the MBRRACE UK 2009 to 2012 (Knight et al 2014) findings?

Management of uterine rupture

The timing and immediacy of treatment will depend on the maternal and fetal condition. In all cases delivery by caesarean section needs to be expedited and the woman and partner appropriately prepared. In the case of maternal collapse the immediate response is to assess her airway, breathing and circulation and initiate fluid resuscitation. The psychological and emotional effects on the mother and her partner should also be considered, with particular attention to concise and appropriate communication. Once the baby is born the surgeon will assess the damage to the uterus and repair the tear. An artery ligation or hysterectomy may be needed depending on the extent of the bleeding and/or damage.

With a wound dehiscence in a woman having a vaginal birth after caesarean (VBAC), the sequence of events is likely to be less intensive. Fetal distress or slowing of labour may be the only sign that a dehiscence has occurred. The blood loss will also be less owing to the avascular nature of the scar tissue that has opened. The presentation in this type of scenario will depend on whether a small part of the previous wound has opened up or the whole wound site.

Preventing uterine rupture

The key component is careful management of the progress of labour including assessing dilatation of the cervix and descent of the presenting part, and recognizing when labour is abnormal or obstructed. In advanced obstructed labour, an oblique ridge can be seen across the maternal abdomen. This ridge delineates the thick upper uterine segment from the thinned out lower segment. In clinical practice and in medical textbooks this hardened abnormal ridge is sometimes referred to as Bandl's ring, named after the Viennese obstetrician Ludwig Bandl. If this situation occurs, the lower segment will be dangerously thinned and there is a high risk of uterine rupture. Such a presentation of obstructed labour is rare in the UK, whereas in developing countries with limited medical aid this is more common (Oyston et al 2014).

The midwife also needs to consider and determine why labour has slowed: it may be due to a mal-presentation, a degree of cephalo-pelvic disproportion or inadequate uterine contractions. Assessing these factors is important, as they will inform the management plan and whether or not it is safe to introduce an oxytocin infusion to augment labour.

The use of an oxytocin infusion should follow a set local guideline, with the infusion gradually increased over time. The midwife must be vigilant for overstimulation of the uterus, and she will need to palpate the contractions if the woman has an epidural and not rely solely on the Toco readings of the cardiotocograph. As discussed earlier, misuse of oxytocin is a major factor in uterine rupture (Knight et al 2014). In the event of hyperstimulation, the oxytocin infusion should be stopped and the use of a tocolytic such as terbutaline considered.

Activity

Reflect on the findings of the MMBRACE report and think about how often you have cared for someone with a syntocinon infusion. How confident do you feel palpating and assessing contractions when a woman has an epidural?

Vaginal birth after caesarean

A woman planning to have a vaginal birth after a primary caesarean will already be aware that she has a slightly higher chance of uterine rupture. However, it is useful to help the woman put this in context. The risk of a delivery-related perinatal death is 0.04% (Royal College of Obstetricians and Gynaecologists (RCOG) 2015), and this is the same as the risk for a first-time mother giving birth. Also, labour progress is monitored very carefully with early recourse for a caesarean section if it is considered the safest option for mother and/or baby. The other two main recommendations are that women give birth in hospital with close availability of appropriate personnel and also that continuous monitoring is used throughout the labour as an early warning sign for wound dehiscence or pending rupture.

The use of prostaglandins to induce labour increases the risk of uterine rupture to 3.0 per 1000, and when labour is also augmented the risk rises to 3.6 per 1000. This is in comparison to a rate of 1.3 per 1000 if no prostaglandin is used to induce and no subsequent augmentation is used during labour (Fitzpatrick et al 2012). In most cases induction is not contraindicated; however, it must be managed carefully and any other risk factors taken into consideration (RCOG 2015).

Activity

Look at your hospital guideline for the use of oxytocin to augment labour. Does it make distinctions between grand multiparous and nulliparous women? Does it recommend oxytocin augmentation for multiparous women in the second stage of labour?

Uterine inversion

Uterine inversion (Fig. 9.1) occurs after the baby is born and is usually associated with the management of the third stage or labour. It is less common than a ruptured uterus, though accurate incidence rates are difficult to quantify, with ranges from 1 : 2000 to 1 : 23,000 quoted (O'Grady 2008; Bhalla et al 2009).

The term uterine inversion applies to the fundus inverting and collapsing down into the uterus as it protrudes downwards. In a partial inversion the fundus does not pass through the cervix; in more serious cases the fundus can protrude through the cervix and may appear outside of the vagina. Owing to the rapid access to treatment in the developed world, maternal death from uterine inversion is rare.

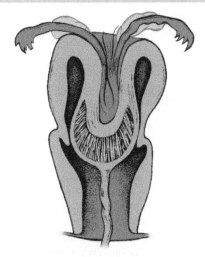

Fig. 9.1 Inversion of gravid uterus. (With permission from Macdonald S, Johnson G, eds., Mayes' Midwifery, 15th ed., p. 1102, Fig. 67.7. Oxford: Elsevier.)

Risk factors

The most commonly cited risk factor is mismanagement of the third stage of labour. This may involve fundal pressure or, more commonly, excessive pulling of the cord to a fundally implanted placenta that has not completely separated (Baskett et al 2007).

Other risk factors cited include:

+ Macrosomia
+ Short cord
+ Morbidly adherent placenta
+ Precipate labour
+ Maternal structural disorders
+ Disorder involving connective tissue

In 50% of cases no predisposing risk factors will be present (Adesiyun 2007).

Symptoms

+ Pale and sweaty maternal appearance
+ Maternal hypotension
+ Neurogenic and/or cardiovascular shock
+ Pain
+ Haemorrhage

- Inverted fundus felt in the vagina
- Inverted fundus seen at introitus

Activity

In terms of managing the third stage of labour safely, what do you know about the term 'guarding the uterus' and is there any evidence to show this is beneficial/important?

Management

First-line management includes immediate treatment of shock (see Chapter 1) and immediate replacement of the inverted uterus. How the uterus is repositioned will depend on the maternal condition and the degree of inversion. If the placenta is still attached it will be left, as attempted removal may lead to extensive haemorrhage. The uterus must be replaced quickly to avoid further trauma and shock. The immediacy of management that is required may limit options for pain relief initially. With manual replacement the delivery bed is elevated at the foot end and manual replacement done by the obstetrician by pushing the inverted fundus back through and up while also applying pressure abdominally. Once the uterus is back in place an oxytocin infusion is started to stimulate the uterus to contract.

Another method practised in the UK is repositioning of the uterus by hydrostatic pressure (Tower 2011). This is usually performed in theatre under a general anaesthetic and involves a silastic ventouse cup being placed in the vagina; a large-bore giving set is then attached and warm saline introduced into the upper vagina by gravity. The fundus is then repositioned as a result of the hydrostatic pressure. If these attempts fail a laparotomy may be performed to surgically correct the inversion.

Activity

What equipment is available in your maternity unit to deal with an acute uterine inversion and how accessible is it?

Preventing an inverted uterus

Prevention may not be possible in all cases, for example with an abnormally adherent fundally placed placenta. However, careful management of the third stage of labour is key, and this includes applying appropriate force during downward traction and early recognition of a problem.

REFLECTION ON THE TRIGGER SCENARIO

Look back on the trigger scenario at the start of the chapter.

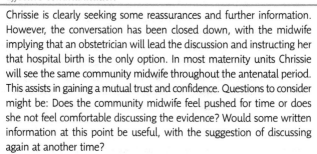

Chrissie is expecting her second child and is anxious about giving birth again, as her first child was born by caesarean section after a long labour. At the booking appointment she asks her community midwife if she will be OK this time and if she can try again for a homebirth. Her midwife tells her that there is a risk of scar rupture and that she must give birth in a hospital; she reassures her that an obstetrician will discuss it all with her at the hospital and if she wants she could just have a repeat caesarean. Afterwards the community midwife says to her student midwife, 'Once you have seen a rupture it makes you really cautious.'

Now that you have an awareness of the evidence surrounding uterine rupture you should have insight into how the scenario relates to the issues involved. The jigsaw model will now be used to explore the trigger scenario in more depth.

Effective communication

Chrissie is clearly seeking some reassurances and further information. However, the conversation has been closed down, with the midwife implying that an obstetrician will lead the discussion and instructing her that hospital birth is the only option. In most maternity units Chrissie will see the same community midwife throughout the antenatal period. This assists in gaining a mutual trust and confidence. Questions to consider might be: Does the community midwife feel pushed for time or does she not feel comfortable discussing the evidence? Would some written information at this point be useful, with the suggestion of discussing again at another time?

Woman-centred care

When women have had a previous caesarean section, maternity guidelines can appear to limit maternal choice. Chrissie may be worried about how her labour will be managed this time; she may just want some reassurances that she *can* labour again and that there is nothing inherently wrong with her body. Questions to ponder would be: How much of the midwife's response is ingrained in her own fear or culturally accepted practices and routines? How do you think the midwife could have better facilitated decision making in this booking interview? When midwives talk about women-centred care does it apply only to women who are low risk?

Using best evidence

In this scenario the community midwife appears to be hesitant about the value of a vaginal birth for Chrissie. Understanding the evidence base is vital to be able to support women during pregnancy. Although a home birth may not be recommended, the evidence could be applied to facilitating a positive hospital birth. The use of mobile telemetry is now widespread in maternity units and a calm environment should not be limited to home birth. In this scenario the community midwife seems to have a negative view of vaginal birth after caesarean. Putting risk in context and using it alongside best evidence and maternal wishes can facilitate a safe and positive experience. How much of this evidence does the community midwife feel comfortable discussing? What else do you think might be influencing the midwife's response in this scenario? Considering the RCOG (2015) 72% to 75% success rate for VBAC, how does your maternity unit compare and how widely are the data shared?

Professional and legal issues

The Nursing and Midwifery Council (NMC) code (2015) states that midwives must *listen to people and respond to their preferences and concerns*. It also states that midwives must *practice in line with best available evidence*. Midwives also have a professional responsibility in terms of public health and in ensuring women and newborns have the best start to their relationship. This includes ensuring intervention in childbirth is discussed with the woman and that she understands the implications of declining or accepting a particular course of action. When would be the most appropriate time to discuss Chrissie's birth plans? What is the best way to document the discussions that take place between Chrissie and the midwife?

Team working

For women with a previous caesarean section, obstetric involvement antenatally is standard in UK maternity units. For the majority of women vaginal birth will be recommended, although it is still often referred to as a 'trial of labour'. How much of a team approach is reflected in this scenario? A question to consider might be: Does the midwife feel her role is undermined by an obstetrician being the lead professional for care? Thinking about this scenario, what might be the benefit of a midwife leading this discussion rather than obstetrician? How can a partnership that includes the woman, midwife and obstetrician best be fostered?

Clinical dexterity

The booking assessment requires clinical dexterity to carry out baseline maternal observations and to obtain blood samples. Women who have had a previous caesarean will receive the same level of antenatal care, although, as already discussed, they have different support needs and need additional information. To do this effectively, the midwife needs to be able to respond to Chrissie's questions with confidence, while recognizing when she needs to refer to another professional with enhanced skills in this area. The midwife who cares for Chrissie in labour will need to be able to explain the rationale for electronic fetal monitoring and be able to interpret the cardiotocograph and be alert for potential signs of wound dehiscence.

Models of care

Women with a previous caesarean section scar are usually classified as 'high risk' and therefore need obstetrician-led care rather than midwife-led care. Continuity with a community midwife is also important, including the opportunity to discuss anxieties and plan ahead to birth. Often in a community setting the community midwife will not have access to previous labour notes, so a question to consider might be: Would the availability of previous obstetric records enable the midwife to feel better equipped to discuss vaginal birth after caesarean with Chrissie? It is becoming more common across UK maternity units to set up midwifery-led VBAC clinics. What do you think may be the potential benefits for women, midwives and obstetricians?

Safe environment

It is well recognized that for women who have had a prior caesarean, hospital is the recommended place of birth, as this is considered the safest option. But what about psychological safety? What does Chrissie need in terms of information and reassurance? With a vaginal birth after caesarean the risk to physical safety falls in the intrapartum stage only. In the antenatal period women need good information and support. Chrissie also needs reassurance regarding her ability to give birth again. So when considering a safe environment you might want to ask if all women who have had a prior caesarean need the expertise of a doctor in the antenatal period.

Promotes health

There are considerable health benefits for the mother and baby in avoiding a caesarean section. How the midwife responds to Chrissie's request for information could have a considerable effect on the family unit. Reflect on some of the conversations you have heard regarding VBAC. How positively is vaginal birth discussed by the midwife? How much awareness do you have about the public health issues this scenario raises? Having successive caesareans has an effect on the health of the mother and fetus. Do you think the midwife should discuss family size with Chrissie?

Further scenarios

The following scenarios enable you to consider how specific situations influence the care and advice that the midwife provides. Use the jigsaw model to explore the issues raised in each situation.

SCENARIO 1

Yvonne is 12 weeks into her third pregnancy. Her first baby was born vaginally and her second baby via an elective caesarean section for breech presentation. Yvonne is unsure what to do this time and asks her community midwife for advice.

Practice point

Women often need time to discuss previous birth experiences in the antenatal period. Yvonne has had two very different births and it would be useful to understand her appraisal of each one. For women who have had a vaginal birth before, the success rate of VBAC increases. Assessing Yvonne's awareness and knowledge of VBAC will be an important element of care.

Further questions may be:
+ What evidence will the community midwife use to discuss VBAC with Yvonne?
+ What might be important to Yvonne when thinking about which type of birth to choose?
+ What might Yvonne already know about VBAC?
+ How might size of family influence the discussion?
+ If this baby is also breech at term, will that alter Yvonne's options?

SCENARIO 2

Jill is 10 days postnatal and wants to understand what happened in labour, as she found her birth experience very upsetting. She gave birth to her fourth child vaginally but there was a problem with getting the placenta out, and her understanding is that the midwife pulled too hard and dislodged her womb.

Practice point

Sometimes women have a limited understanding of human physiology and anatomy. In this type of scenario, using an illustration to increase Jill's understanding may be useful. Just taking time to listen to how she feels is also important. Uterine inversion is a rare event, so it may be that it would beneficial for her to talk to an obstetrician also, especially if she has questions about future births. Although women are often debriefed in the immediate postnatal period, they are often unable to process and/or remember the information so soon after a dramatic event.

Further questions may be:

+ What information can Jill recall being given during her stay in hospital?
+ How was Jill's inversion managed and what type of inversion was it?
+ What is Jill's obstetric history, in particular, mode of birth and any history of problems with the third stage?
+ What does Jill understand about how an inversion occurs?
+ How is Jill feeling emotionally as she processes the information?

Conclusion

Although the incidence of uterine emergencies is relatively low, their effect can be life threatening. The midwife needs to be able to talk to women about their obstetric history and how this might influence the choice of care pathway that best meets their needs. To provide personalized, evidence-based care the midwife must keep up-to-date with the current national guidance and learning from confidential enquiries and professional debate.

Resources
Good review of the evidence
Vadeboncoeur, H., 2011. Birthing Normally After a Caesarean or Two: A guide for Pregnant Women, Exploring Reasons and Practibilities for VBAC, second ed. Fresh Heart Publishing. paperback.
Innovative practice, to increase VBAC uptake
White, H., May, A., Cluett, E., 2016. Evaluating a midwife led model of antenatal care for women with a previous caesarean section: a retrospective, comparative cohort study. Birth 43, 200–208.
The language of risk
Coxon, K., Homer, C., Bisits, A., et al., 2016. Reconceptualising risk in childbirth. Midwifery 38, 1–5.

References
Adesiyun, A.G., 2007. Septic postpartum uterine inversion. Singapore Med. J. 48, 943–945.
Baskett, T.F., Calder, A.A., Arulkumaran, S. (Eds.), 2007. Acute uterine inversion. In: Munro Kerr's Operative Obstetrics, Eleventh ed. Elsevier, London, pp. 243–249.
Bhalla, R., Wuntakal, R., Odejinmi, F., et al., 2009. Acute inversion of the uterus. TOG 11, 13–18.

Fitzpatrick, K.E., Kurinczuk, J.J., Alfirevic, Z., et al., 2012. Uterine rupture by intended mode of delivery in the UK: a national case-control study. PLoS Med. 9, e1001184.

Knight, M., Kenyon, S., Brocklehurst, P., et al. on behalf of MBRRACE-UK, 2014. Saving lives, Improving Mothers' Care: Lessons Learned to Inform Future Maternity Care From the UK and Ireland Confidential Enquiries into Maternal Deaths and Morbidity 2009–12. National Perinatal Epidemiology Unit, University of Oxford, Oxford.

Nursing and Midwifery Council (NMC). 2015. The code: professional standards of practice and behaviour for nurses and midwives. Available at: https://www.nmc.org.uk/globalassets/sitedocuments/nmc-publications/nmc-code.pdf.

O'Grady, J.P., 2008. Malposition of the uterus. eMedicine 272, 497.

Oyston, C., Rueda-Clausen, C.F., Baker, P.N., 2014. Current challenges in pregnancy-related mortality. Obstet. Gynaecol. Reprod. Med. 24, 162–169.

Royal College of Obstetricians and Gynaecologists (RCOG). 2015 Birth after previous caesarean birth (Green-top Guideline 45). https://www.rcog.org.uk/globalassets/documents/guidelines/gtg_45.pdf.

Tahseen, S., Griffiths, M., 2010. Vaginal birth after two caesarean sections (VBAC-2)—a systematic review with meta-analysis of success rate and adverse outcomes of VBAC-2 versus VBAC- 1 and repeat (third) caesarean sections. BJOG 117, 5–19.

Tower, C., 2011. Obstetric emergencies. In: Baker, P., Kenny, L. (Eds.), Obstetrics by Ten Teachers, nineteenth ed. Hodder Arnold, London.

CHAPTER 10

Cord complications

Cord compression, cord presentation, cord prolapse

Alison Brodrick

TRIGGER SCENARIO

Jane is expecting her fifth baby and has now reached 39 weeks' gestation. She has been admitted at night to the antenatal ward with an unstable lie and mild contractions. Her other children were born vaginally without complications. Jane has not slept all night; the contractions have now stopped but her waters have just broken. She informs the midwife, who immediately commences cardiotocography. There is fetal bradycardia and the midwife calls for help. Jane can see from the midwife's panicked look that something is wrong and asks for her husband to be called. Suddenly there are lots of doctors and midwives at her bedside.

Introduction

An umbilical cord event is often sudden and unexpected. However, there are times when the risk of a possible cord accident is increased and actions can be taken to minimize such an occurrence or ensure it is diagnosed quickly. The umbilical cord is vital for transporting oxygenated blood to the fetus. Any interruption to this function of the umbilical cord during pregnancy or labour will therefore reduce blood flow and may lead to fetal compromise.

Cord compression

The most common cord event that can interrupt blood supply to the fetus is cord compression. This is usually evident during labour. It occurs as a result of the cord being squeezed during a contraction, leading to a brief interruption of the fetal blood supply. It usually presents with variable decelerations evident on the cardiotocograph (CTG) with some or all contractions (Gibb 2008). In a healthy term infant with the reserves to cope with the stresses of labour, it is usually safe to continue unless there are further concerns about fetal well-being. Sometimes the compression can be caused by the presenting part as it descends and pushes against the cord or when the cord is wrapped around the neck, body or limb of the fetus (Van der Hout-Van der Jagt et al 2013).

Cord presentation and cord prolapse

Unlike cord compression during labour, cord presentation and cord prolapse are less common but present an increased risk to the fetus (Arulkumaran 2013).

Cord presentation can occur in pregnancy and/or in labour and is the term used when the fetal membranes are intact, and, as the name suggests, the cord lies in front of the fetal presenting part. The term 'occult cord' refers to the cord lying alongside the fetal presenting part (Lin 2006). In most cases cord presentation goes undetected (Oats & Abraham 2010) until the fetal membranes break and the cord presentation is then termed 'cord prolapse'. When this occurs, the risk of fetal compromise is high and delivery must be expedited.

Risk factors

The risk factors for both cord presentation and cord prolapse are the same (see Box 10.1). Any situation in which the presenting part is displaced or is not well applied to the cervix will increase the risk that a loop of cord can drop in front of the fetal presenting part (Arulkumaran 2013).

Approximately 50% of cases occur as a result of an intervention or procedure (Usta et al 1999). These main causes are:

+ External cephalic version
+ Internal podalic version
+ Artificial rupture of membranes (ARM) with a high presenting part

Reducing the risk of cord prolapse

Clinicians should be aware of the risk factors for cord prolapse and be vigilant to ensure appropriate management of pregnancy and labour so as to not increase the risk of a prolapse occurring. In the UK a woman who has an unstable, transverse or oblique lie at term will often warrant inpatient

---

Box 10.1 **Risk factors for cord presentation and cord prolapse**

High head or ill-fitting presenting part
Transverse, oblique and unstable lie
Mal-presentation, especially breech
Multiple pregnancy
Multiparity
Prematurity
Polyhydramnios
Low-lying placenta
Small or growth-restricted baby
Fetal congenital anomalies
(RCOG 2014)

admission (Royal College of Obstetricians and Gynaecologists (RCOG) 2014). Although this does not reduce the risk of a cord prolapse occurring, it does reduce the time taken to diagnose and treat cord prolapse when it occurs (Lin 2006). The management will then be dependent on the individual clinical history but may include an external cephalic version and immediate induction of labour if a cephalic presentation can be maintained. All women with a mal-presentation including breech presentation should be informed of the need to seek immediate hospital assessment if spontaneous rupture of the membranes occurs.

Interventions that should be avoided include ARM when there is a high presenting part or if a cord presentation is felt on vaginal examination. It is possible to perform ARM with a high head but this is usually done in theatre (RCOG 2014), with the ability to proceed straight to caesarean if a prolapse occurs. In these cases the potential for a poor outcome is assessed alongside potential benefits of performing the intervention (Chebsey et al 2012). If a cord presentation is suspected in labour then an emergency caesarean is usually indicated.

Incidence

The overall incidence rate of umbilical cord prolapse ranges from 0.1% to 0.6% (RCOG 2014), but in breech presentation the incidence of cord prolapse is higher, at 1% (Panter & Hannah 1996). There is evidence, however, that the rate has declined considerably over time. Retrospective data from Dublin demonstrate a rate of 6.4 per 1000 live births in the 1940s to 1.7 per 1000 in the 2000s (Gibbons et al 2014). This change is largely attributed to the reduction in grand multiparity, which in the 1940s accounted for 75% of cases. Perinatal survival has also improved; with better management, awareness and fetal surveillance the chance of survival has increased from 46% in the 1940s to 96% in the 21st century (Gibbons et al 2014).

Clinical presentation

A cord presentation can be diagnosed when a vaginal examination is performed and the pulsating cord is felt at the same rate as the fetal heart through the membranes. It can also be suspected if there is a suspicious CTG pattern. It is also possible on occasion to diagnose during ultrasound scan, but this is not considered a reliable diagnostic or screening tool in terms of avoiding prolapse and/or improving fetal outcome (Kinugasa et al 2007). There is some benefit in using ultrasound to diagnose cord presentation with a breech presentation to inform mode of birth (RCOG 2014).

A cord prolapse can be diagnosed in three ways (see Box 10.2).

Box 10.2 **Diagnosis of cord prolapse**

> ***See it*** – when it protrudes outside of the body
> ***Hear it*** – bradycardia or variable decelerations
> ***Feel it*** – during a vaginal examination

Box 10.3 **Relieving cord compression**

> Digitally pushing the presenting part upwards
> Maternal position – all-fours/knee-to-chest; exaggerated Sim's
> Maternal bladder filling

The change in pressure as the waters break can result in the cord being expelled quickly past the presenting part, through the cervix and out through the introitus. There is a high risk of this occurring in the presence of poly-hydramnios and an ill-fitting presenting part. In these circumstances, a prolapse is easy to diagnose (*See it*). When a cord prolapse occurs cord compression can occur as the fetal presenting part follows the cord downwards and rests on the cord. In this scenario the cord prolapse can be diagnosed by a change in fetal heart please read continuing text (*Hear it*); depending on the degree of compression this could be a bradycardia or more commonly variable decelerations (RCOG 2014). A cord prolapse is also diagnosed during a vaginal examination when the cord is felt pulsating during the examination (*Feel it*). Cord prolapse can occur with no outward physical signs or changes to the fetal heart and diagnosed only when a routine vaginal examination is performed (Chebsey et al 2012). When a cord prolapse is diagnosed there should minimal handing of the cord to prevent vasospasm (RCOG 2014) and fetal compromise as the blood supply is further restricted.

Management of cord prolapse

If the prolapse occurs before full dilatation, then the woman and her partner must be prepared for an immediate caesarean section, as the risk of fetal compromise is high.

While preparations are initiated for delivery, immediate management should aim to relieve the cord compression. This can be achieved in a number of ways (see Box 10.3):

• Digitally pushing the presenting part upwards (Fig. 10.1)

When a cord prolapse has been diagnosed during a vaginal examination, the attending clinician should leave his or her hand in situ, and using two fingers manually push the presenting part upwards.

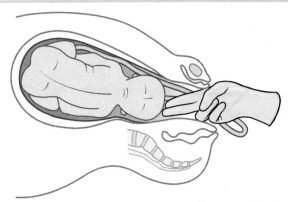

Fig. 10.1 Displacement of the presenting part. (With permission from Goonwardene M. Umbilical cord propalse. In: Chandraharan E, Arulkumaran S, eds., Obstetric and Intrapartum Emergencies: A Practical Guide to Management. Cambridge: Cambridge University Press.)

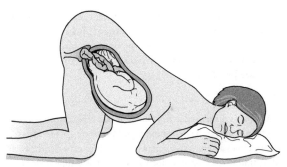

Fig. 10.2 Knee-to-chest position. (With permission from Marshall J, Raynor M, eds., Myles Textbook for Midwives, 16th ed., p. 478, Fig. 22.2. Edinburgh: Churchill Livingstone/Elsevier.)

- Maternal position: all-fours/knee-to-chest (Fig. 10.2)
- Exaggerated Sim's position (Fig. 10.3)

Compression can be further minimized by supporting the woman into either an all-fours position and then adopting a knee-to-chest position or left lateral with a head-down tilt and a pillow used to elevate the hips (also known as exaggerated Sim's) (RCOG 2014; Chebsey et al 2012).

- Maternal bladder filling

Another method of relieving cord compression is to fill the bladder with water (Vago 1970). As the bladder inflates, the presenting part is displaced,

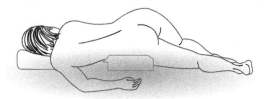

Fig. 10.3 Exaggerated Sim's position. (With permission from Macdonald S, Johnson G, eds., Mayes' Midwifery, 15th ed., p. 1076, Fig. 65.3. Oxford: Elsevier.)

Box 10.4 **Bladder filling to relieve cord compression**

> Pass a 16G Foley catheter and drain the bladder.
> Attach a blood giving set to the Foley catheter.
> Free flow 500 to 750 ml of warm normal saline.
> Remove the giving set and place a spigot in the end of the Foley catheter.

relieving cord compression. This is useful when there is a risk that delivery will be delayed, for instance, in a community setting (Chebsey et al 2012). For this reason it is recommended that all community midwives carry the equipment needed to fill the bladder (RCOG 2014) and are familiar with the procedure (see Box 10.4).

Management of cord prolapse in the second stage of labour

If the cord prolapse is diagnosed at full dilatation in a cephalic presentation, it is possible that birth can be expedited with forceps or a ventouse, or in a multiparous woman an episiotomy may be enough to expedite the birth. When birth is imminent outcomes for vaginal birth are similar or better than for a caesarean section (Murphy & MacKenzie 1995).

Whenever a cord prolapse is diagnosed, an immediate and appropriate response from the entire maternity team is needed. Ensuring teams work effectively is essential for management of all obstetric emergencies; in the case of cord prolapse annual multidisciplinary training has been shown to improve the diagnosis to delivery interval (Siassakos et al 2009). During simulated training, it is important that the role of supporting the mother and partner is also acknowledged. Any potentially life-threatening event can evoke feelings of heightened fear, leading to psychological problems, even if actions are timely and the outcome good (Vincent 2006). To promote positive mental health after the event, having a reassuring clinician who can provide tactile contact and explain what is happening is important (Mapp & Hudson 2005).

Jane is expecting her fifth baby and has now reached 39 weeks' gestation. She has been admitted at night to the antenatal ward with an unstable lie and mild contractions. Her other children were born vaginally without complications. Jane has not slept all night; the contractions have now stopped but her waters have just broken. She informs the midwife, who immediately commences cardiotocography. There is fetal bradycardia and the midwife calls for help. Jane can see from the midwife's panicked look that something is wrong and asks for her husband to be called. Suddenly there are lots of doctors and midwives at her bedside.

Now that you have an awareness of the evidence surrounding cord emergencies you should have insight into how the scenario relates to the issues involved. The jigsaw model will now be used to explore the trigger scenario in more depth.

Effective communication

Jane is likely to be feeling anxious and fearful. Her previous births were uncomplicated and this may be the first time she has been admitted to hospital. There is already some non-verbal communication occurring, as Jane has picked up on the midwife's facial expression. Jane has asked for her husband to be called, but this request may be lost as events move quickly. In this scenario effective, concise and accurate communication is an important element of appropriate management. The midwife has just arrived on duty and is going to need to communicate effectively to the multidisciplinary team as they arrive. If the midwife has just arrived on duty she may not have had a full handover or may not have retained all the information. Questions to consider might be: What does Jane already understand about her reason for admission and the possible consequences? How might the team communicate with Jane while also assessing the clinical picture? The handover process is a key element in ensuring safe and timely care. How might the midwife access the information she needs quickly?

Woman-centred care

With an antenatal admission of this kind it is easy to see how the principles of *woman-centred care* can be lost owing to the need to deal with the sudden emergency. Information giving in this type of scenario is very important to enable women to feel safe. Questions to ask might be: Who is best placed to reassure Jane and provide some information? Has someone organized for her husband to be called? Jane has had experience only of vaginal births. If the cervix is not fully dilated and a cord prolapse is diagnosed, an emergency caesarean will be necessary. How should this be addressed by the team providing care?

Using best evidence

When the clinicians arrive at Jane's bedside the first thing they will see and hear is the bradycardia. The midwife may have already moved Jane into a left lateral position to optimize blood supply to the fetus. If the bradycardia continues, National Institute for Health and Care Excellence (NICE) guidance on fetal monitoring (NICE 2017) recommends preparing for theatre. As the clinicians become aware of Jane's clinical history and reason for admission, assessing for cord prolapse via a vaginal examination will determine further management. Questions to consider might be: Does the antenatal ward have bladder-filling equipment if needed? Although elevating the presenting part is best practice with a cord prolapse, what challenges may this pose on an antenatal ward?

Professional and legal issues

The Nursing and Midwifery Council (NMC) code (2015) states that registrants must *listen to people and respond to their preferences and concerns*. It also states that midwives must *practice in line with best available evidence*. The midwife in this scenario should be aware of first-line management in an obstetric emergency. Questions to consider might be: Has the midwife attended a clinical skills training day recently? As a professional registrant, documentation is also important. In this scenario what could be used to assist with timely and concise documentation?

Team working

Teamwork and communication in an emergency situation like this is paramount. The attending clinicians are unlikely to know anything about Jane or her clinical history. Questions to consider might be: Who should assume control and lead the management? How far is the antenatal ward from the labour ward and how will this affect how the team responds and acts? In an emergency it is important that accurate records and timings of personnel attending and interventions performed are maintained. Who might be best placed in the team to record activity and timings?

Clinical dexterity

The midwife responds to Jane's history with prompt clinical action. She hears a fetal bradycardia and alerts the maternity care team without delay. With a cord prolapse, time is of the essence. The generally accepted first line of management is to perform a vaginal examination and push the presenting part upwards, though the majority of midwives will have done this only in a simulated environment. Questions to ponder would be: what training or experience is the midwife likely to have had in dealing with a cord presentation and how might this affect how she responds? What might be the effect on the midwife undertaking this procedure? Consider how the midwife will be positioned during the trip to theatre.

Models of care

Jane has previously been under a midwife led model of care, her previous births were uncomplicated and it may be that she had no obstetric input. With an unstable lie and possible cord prolapse she now requires immediate obstetric support and faces potential surgical intervention. It is likely that Jane will now have a team of clinicians looking after her including anaesthetists, obstetricians and midwives. How each one deals with and acts within this situation will affect how Jane remembers her care. Questions to consider might be: How might this sudden unplanned situation affect Jane and what could be done to reduce her anxiety now and in the postnatal period?

Safe environment

It is important that Jane feels psychologically and physically safe. Jane is on an antenatal ward and may be in a bay with other pregnant women. Questions to consider might be: How can Jane's privacy and dignity be maintained? How might the other women on the ward be feeling and what could be done to alleviate their anxiety?

Promotes health

Jane has not experienced problems in her other pregnancies and births. With younger children at home, being in hospital could be adding considerable stress to Jane. What is the potential effect of a stress response in pregnancy potential on the fetus? Feeling in control is well acknowledged in maternity care and plays a big part in how women appraise their situation. How do you think Jane is feeling at the moment and how might that manifest in her behaviour?

Further scenarios

The following scenarios enable you to consider how specific situations influence the care and advise that the midwife provides. Use the jigsaw model to explore the issues raised in each situation.

SCENARIO 1

Karen is 36 weeks pregnant and is feeling increasingly anxious about labour and particularly her waters breaking. In her last pregnancy, she had a cord prolapse and found the situation very upsetting.

Practice point

Although women are often debriefed in the immediate postnatal period, they are often unable to process and/or remember the information so soon after a dramatic event. As healthcare professionals, we see a cord prolapse as a rare event. Many midwives will go a whole career without having to deal with such an event. For a woman, however, the fear of a prolapse occurring again usually remains high until her baby has safely arrived. When an untoward event has occurred in a previous pregnancy or previous labour women often want that information to be easily visible to the attending clinicians in the hospital so that it is acknowledged as part of the clinical plan.

Further questions may be:

- What is Karen's obstetric history, and does this influence the mode of birth this time?
- What does Karen understand about what happened last time?
- What are the circumstances that led to the cord prolapse and how easy it is for the community midwife to get this information?
- What else could be put in place to ensure Karen feels more secure?

SCENARIO 2

Hannah has been admitted for an induction of labour at term. On palpation the head is high and not fixed in the pelvis. This is her second baby. She has been waiting for her induction for more than 24 hours, and with childcare now rearranged is keen for the induction to go ahead straightaway.

Practice point

In this scenario a vaginal examination is likely to follow after abdominal palpation. The vaginal examination will enable the clinician to assess the cervix. The decision to administer a cervical ripening agent is a different consideration from planning an ARM. The other factors will be dependent on the obstetric history and reason for induction. If appropriate a 'controlled' rupture of membranes can be considered, but this needs to be carefully communicated to the woman and her partner.

Further questions may be:

+ What other information is needed before a further plan can be made?
+ What might be the reason for a high head at term in a multiparous woman?
+ How can information be delivered to Hannah and her partner without causing undue alarm?
+ Where is Hannah being cared for currently, and will this affect the plan?
+ Who should be involved in a 'controlled' rupture of membranes and in what environment?

Conclusion

Cord emergencies are rare events that require an immediate and appropriate response from clinicians. Team working and communication are vital and all maternity staff should be involved in regular simulated training. Clinicians must be aware of maternal/fetal circumstances that increase the risk of cord prolapse and also their own clinical interventions that may also increase the risk. Women need time to process events and to understand the implications for a next pregnancy and birth.

Resources
Importance of training
See Siasskos et al in the reference list that follows and also:

Copson, S., Calvert, K., Raman, P., et al., 2017. The effect of a multidisciplinary obstetric emergency team training program, the In Time course, on diagnosis to delivery interval following umbilical cord prolapse – a retrospective cohort study. Aust. N. Z. J. Obstet. Gynaecol. 57, 327–333.

Bladder filling
Houghton, G., 2006. Bladder filling: an effective technique for managing cord prolapse. Br. J. Midwifery 14, 88–89.

Patient information leaflet
RCOG, 2015. Umbilical cord prolapse in later pregnancy. Available at: https://www.rcog.org.uk/en/patients/patient-leaflets/umbilical-cord-prolapse-in-late-pregnancy/.

References
Arulkumaran, S., 2013. Management of labour. In: Symonds, M. (Ed.), Essential Obstetrics and Gynaecology, fifth ed. Churchill Livingstone, Edinburgh.

Chebsey, C., Siassakos, D., Draycott, T., 2012. A review of umbilical cord prolapse and the influence of training on management. Fetal Matern. Med. Rev. 23, 120–130.

Gibb, D.M., 2008. Fetal Monitoring in Practice, third ed. Butterworth Heinemann, Edinburgh.

Gibbons, C., OHerlihy, C., Murphy, J.F., 2014. Umbilical cord prolapse: changing patterns and improved outcomes. BJOG 121, 1705–1709.

Kinugasa, M., Sato, T., Tamura, M., et al., 2007. Antepartum detection of cord presentation by transvaginal ultrasonography for term breech presentation: potential prediction and prevention of cord prolapse. J. Obstet. Gynaecol. Res. 33, 612–618.

Lin, M.G., 2006. Umbilical cord prolapse. Obstet. Gynecol. Surv. 61, 269–277.

Mapp, T., Hudson, K., 2005. Feelings and fears during obstetric emergencies. Br. J. Midwifery 13, 1.

Murphy, D.J., MacKenzie, I.Z., 1995. The mortality and morbidity associated with umbilical cord prolapse. Br. J. Obstet. Gynaecol. 102, 826–830.

National Institute Health and Care Excellence (NICE), 2017. Intrapartum Care for healthy women and babies. NICE London.

Oats, J., Abraham, S. (Eds.), 2010. Llewellyn–Jones Fundamentals of Obstetrics and Gynaecology, ninth ed. Mosby Elsevier, St. Louis.

Panter, K.R., Hannah, M.E., 1996. Umbilical cord prolapse: so far so good? Lancet 347, 74.

RCOG, 2014. Umbilical Cord Prolapse. Green Top Guideline No 50. RCOG London. https://www.rcog.org.uk/globalassets/documents/guidelines/gtg-50 -umbilicalcordprolapse-2014.pdf.

Siassakos, D., Hasafa, Z., Sibanda, T., 2009. Retrospective cohort study of diagnosis–delivery interval with umbilical cord prolapse: the effect of team training. BJOG 116, 1089–1096.

Usta, I.M., Mercer, B.M., Sibai, B.M., 1999. Current obstetrical practice and umbilical cord prolapse. Am. J. Perinatol. 16, 479–484.

Vago, T., 1970. Prolapse of the umbilical cord: a method of management. Am. J. Obstet. Gynecol. 107, 967–969.

Van der Hout-Van der Jagt, M.B., Jongen, G.J., Bovendeerd, P.H., Oei, S.G., 2013. Insight into variable fetal heart rate decelerations from a mathematical model. Early Hum. Dev. 89, 361–369.

Vincent, C., 2006. Patient Safety. Churchill Livingstone, Edinburgh.

CHAPTER 11

Maternal sepsis

TRIGGER SCENARIO

Julie phoned labour ward triage complaining of abdominal pain and just not feeling well. She was 28 weeks pregnant, expecting her first baby. Kim, the midwife, ran through the routine questions, 'Have you had any bleeding, any loss of fluid…?' Julie said that she thought she had leaked some urine 3 days ago and had felt damp ever since, but thought that was because the baby was pressing on her bladder. Kim said, 'I want you to make your way into the unit so we can check you and your baby over'.

Introduction

Sepsis is a serious and life-threatening condition that can rapidly overwhelm a woman's defenses, leading to death or serious morbidity, and is the leading cause of maternal death worldwide (Say et al 2014). It is estimated that 44,000 people in the UK die of sepsis (UK Sepsis Trust 2018), yet if detected early, it can have very good outcomes. The number of maternal deaths due to sepsis has declined in recent Confidential Enquiries (Knight et al 2016, 2017) thought to be influenced by increased awareness of this deadly condition. This chapter explores the common causes of sepsis in the childbearing woman and how it can be recognized and treated.

Definition

Sepsis is defined as:

> 'a life-threatening organ dysfunction due to a dysregulated host response to infection' (NICE 2016, 2017)
>> and
> 'the presence of an infection with the manifestations of a systemic inflammatory response (SIRS)'

(Knight et al 2014: 28)

Put simply, sepsis happens when a person's body reacts to an infection in such a way that it leads to organ and tissue damage. Sepsis may also be known as 'blood poisoning' or 'septicaemia'.

Box 11.1 **Recommendations from MBRRACE report (2017)**

1. Those carrying out postnatal checks in the community should have a thermometer to check the temperature of a woman who feels unwell.
2. When assessing a woman who is unwell, consider her clinical condition in addition to her MEOWS score.
3. Consider 'declaring sepsis' to activate a protocol that informs the multi-professional team so they are ready to act.
4. Within 24 hours of giving birth women should be aware of the signs of life-threatening conditions so they know when to seek urgent help.

The incidence of maternal sepsis has been reported to be 0.1% to 0.3% in developed countries and the risk doubles when labour starts and increases threefold postnatally (Knowles et al 2015).

Prevention

The best way to prevent the body from responding adversely to an infection is to prevent infection from developing in the first place. According to the World Health Organisation (WHO 2017), most infections can be prevented through access to immunization and improved hygiene.

An important turning point in reducing the prevalence of maternal sepsis in England came after the 2009 to 2012 Confidential Enquiries into Maternal Deaths (Knight et al 2014). Acting on the tragic loss of 83 women to overwhelming infection, the report urged healthcare professionals to 'think sepsis' when caring for an unwell pregnant or recently pregnant woman. Of the 83 women, 36 died from influenza at the time of the H1N1 influenza pandemic. A subsequent public health campaign to promote the uptake of the seasonal flu vaccination has been a huge success and in the 2017 report included only 1 death from flu.

Women should be given information about the sign of life-threatening infection within 24 hours of the birth (Knight et al 2017) and encouraged to use strict hand hygiene at all times, washing their hands before and after going to the toilet. See Box 11.1 for the latest recommendations from MBRRACE (2017).

Activity

Find out what percentage of women in your area access the seasonal flu vaccination.

When is the vaccine offered and by whom? When can the vaccination be given in pregnancy?

Table 11.1: **Risk factors for maternal sepsis**

Life style/ sociodemographics	Medical	Obstetric
Obesity	Anaemia	Caesarean birth
Smoking	Diabetes	Perineal trauma
Drug misuse	Immunosuppressant or steroid therapy	Prolonged rupture of membranes
Age – extremes of	Cuts, burns, skin infections	Retained products of conception
Minority ethnic group	Contact with infectious diseases	Indwelling catheters and lines

Risk factors

Women who are pregnant or have been pregnant in the previous 6 weeks are at high risk for sepsis. This risk is increased if they are unwell, have been subject to invasive procedures or had prolonged rupture of membranes (National Institute for Health and Care Excellence (NICE) 2016, 2017). Other lifestyle factors, such as current smoker, may also add to their risk (see Table 11.1).

Consider sepsis

When a person presents with symptoms of infection and feels unwell, a full set of maternal observations should be made and recorded on a Modified Early Obstetric Warning System (MEOWS) chart. A full clinical history might lead the midwife to go on to *suspect* sepsis, especially when she has one or more of the risk factors listed in Table 11.2.

Suspect sepsis

It is important that criteria for suspecting sepsis are considered so that appropriate investigation and treatment can begin without delay. A bespoke screening tool can assist in this process.

Causes

The actual source of the infection may be readily apparent; for example, if the woman has offensive lochia it is likely to be uterine in origin, perhaps from the placental site or retained products. However, the potential sources are many and may not be obvious. Thus, when a woman is unwell, a detailed history is required to try and identify the source; see Table 11.3 for examples.

Table 11.2: **Risk stratification tool for adults**

Clinical observation	High risk	Moderate to high risk
Systolic blood pressure	90 mm Hg or less, or more than 40 mm Hg below normal for them	91–100 mm Hg
Heart rate	>130 /minute	91–130 beats/minute (100–130 or raise in baseline by 10–15 if pregnant)
Respiratory rate	≥25 breaths/minute	21–24 breaths/minute
Temperature (tympanic)	< 36°C or > 38°C Do not rely on fever or hypothermia to rule sepsis either in or out	
Urine output	Not passed urine in 18 hours <0.5 ml/kg per hour	Not passed urine in 12–18 hours <0.5–1 ml/kg per hour
Mental state	Evidence of new altered mental state Loss of functionality	History of new altered mental health reported by woman or other
Skin	Cyanosis, mottled or ashen nonblanching skin rash	Redness, swelling or discharge at surgical site or wound breakdown

Adapted from NICE (2016, 2017) and RCOG (2012a, 2012b).

Table 11.3: **Sources of infection and associated symptoms**

Source	Detective work: possible symptoms	Tests*
Uterine	Is her uterus tender to the touch? Is her lochia offensive? Was the placenta complete? Did she have prolonged rupture of membranes? Did she have a caesarean section?	Ultrasound for retained products or haematoma. High vaginal/ endocervical/ placental swab
Urinary	Has she been complaining of pain or difficulty passing urine? Is the urine offensive? Has she recently had a urinary catheter? Has she had surgery recently?	Mid-stream specimen of urine (MSU) for culture & sensitivity Catheter specimen of urine Wound swab
Skin	Does she have a perineal or vaginal wound, haematoma? Has she any broken skin, puncture site, spots or boils?	Perineal swab Skin swab

Table 11.3: Sources of infection and associated symptoms (Continued)

Source	Detective work: possible symptoms	Tests*
Breast	Does she have cracked nipples? Has she had mastitis? Are there any red areas, segmentation, pain or inflammation?	Expressed breast milk
Chest	Is she breathless? Does she have a productive cough? Has she had a sore throat recently?	Sputum specimen Chest x-ray study
Gastric	Has she had any recent diarrhoea or vomiting? Has she had any abdominal pain? Is she nauseous?	Stool sample
Brain	Has she any neck stiffness or photophobia? Headache, confusion?	Computerized tomography (CT) scan, lumbar puncture

*All women would have blood taken for culture and sensitivity.

Box 11.2 **Sepsis six**

1. Give oxygen to keep saturation above 94%.
2. Take blood cultures.
3. Give IV antibiotics.
4. Give a fluid challenge.
5. Measure lactate.
6. Measure urine output.

Diagnosis

Confidential Enquiries have advocated that:

> 'where sepsis is suspected a sepsis care bundle must be applied in a structured and systematic way with urgency'
>
> Knight et al (2017: 63)

Application of a sepsis care bundle, such as that advocated by the UK Sepsis Trust, known as the 'Sepsis Six' (see Box 11.2), is recommended. When sepsis has been recognized, the bundle should be implemented within 1 hour (Roberts et al 2017).

Treatment using sepsis six

If at any point during the implementation of a sepsis bundle, the woman's condition deteriorates and she requires resuscitation, the principles of managing maternal collapse, outlined in Chapter 1, should be followed.

1. Oxygen

Oxygen should be given via face mask to achieve saturation of more than 94% to 98% (NICE 2016, 2017).

2. Blood cultures

To inform subsequent treatment, venous blood should be taken for culture and sensitivity, before antibiotics are given. Then IV antibiotics should be given without waiting for the results (see later) (Royal College of Obstetricians and Gynaecologists (RCOG) 2012a, 2012b).

In addition to blood cultures, blood should also be taken for: full blood count (FBC), urea and electrolytes (U&E), glucose and creatinine. Other swabs or specimens may be advocated depending on her history and potential source of infection (see Table 11.3).

Activity

Find out which are the major organisms responsible for sepsis in pregnant or postnatal women.

Find out which antibiotics are used to treat them.

---

3. Antibiotics

Antibiotics should be administered, preferably intravenously, as soon as possible and before culture results are available, to reduce the likelihood of mortality. Choice of antibiotic will depend on current hospital trust policy and always considering any known allergy (UK Sepsis Trust 2016). Ultimately effective treatment for sepsis will be determined by identifying the source and nature of the infection; the results of cultures (blood, urine, sputum and amniotic fluid) will then subsequently inform the choice of antibiotic therapy targeted to the organism(s): goal-directed therapy (Vaught 2018).

Antimicrobial resistance

Although the rapid recourse to intravenous antibiotics is essential when sepsis is suspected, practitioners must be vigilant with their use. Antimicrobial drugs or agents include antibiotics, antivirals and antifungals. They may be naturally occurring or synthetic preparations developed for their therapeutic properties. The use of antibiotics to treat infection has become accepted practice. However, when microorganisms, such as bacteria, viruses and fungi, change after exposure to antibiotics, they can become resistant to the potential life-saving impact of the antimicrobial. This antimicrobial resistance (AMR) has led to the development of 'super bugs', which can be untreatable and lead to a significant consumption of healthcare resources.

Activity

Consider the bacterium methicillin-resistant *Staphylococcus aureus* (MRSA). When is it screened for?

 What care should be given to women who screen positive for MRSA?

---

4. Fluids

Septic shock must be treated with fluid resuscitation. Intravenous fluids are administered while an accurate intake and output record is maintained to ensure that hypervolaemia does not develop with the potential consequence of pulmonary or bowel oedema (Waechter et al 2014). Give a sodium-containing crystalloid as a bolus of 500 millilitres in less than 15 minutes (NICE 2016, 2017). This can be repeated up to 30 ml/kg, and involve anaesthetic input if the woman has pre-eclampsia (UK Sepsis Trust 2016).

5. Lactate

A serum lactate level of 4 mmol/l or greater is indicative of tissue hypoperfusion (RCOG 2012a). Serial lactate should be measured to monitor improvement and after each 10 ml/kg fluid challenge (UK Sepsis Trust 2016). Failure to respond is identified if serum lactate is not reduced by more than 20% within 1 hour (NICE 2016, 2017) and requires consultant input.

6. Urine

Urine output should be measured hourly and recorded on a fluid balance chart (UK Sepsis Trust 2016). Oliguria is diagnosed when output is less than 0.5 ml/kg for at least 2 hours, despite fluid resuscitation (RCOG 2012b). As urine output is a key element of measuring response to treatment, a urinary catheter should be inserted to ensure accurate measurement.

Care of the baby

In the pregnant woman with sepsis, consideration should be given to the best time to deliver the baby and the most appropriate means. Such decisions will be made by a senior obstetrician in consultation with the woman, if possible (RCOG 2012a). Consideration can be given to promoting lung maturity with the use of maternal corticosteroids, although caution should be given, as steroids may suppress the immune response (RCOG 2010). Spinal anaesthesia is contradicted in women with suspected sepsis. Continuous fetal monitoring is recommended for women who have a temperature of 37.5°C on two occasions 1 hour apart or greater than 38°C once (NICE 2014, 2016). After birth the baby should be referred to the care of a neonatologist, for infection screening and possible prophylactic treatment.

Ongoing care

If after the implementation of the Sepsis Six criteria the woman's condition is not improving or her condition is unstable, she should be referred to a critical care facility (UK Sepsis Trust 2016). Meticulous documentation of all actions taken and her response to treatments should be made. Observations should continue on a MEOWS chart to support appropriate and timely escalation where indicated.

A woman with sepsis should be cared for in a single room, and all professionals caring for her should wear appropriate protective clothing (gloves, apron, gown and mask) in line with local infection control guidance. The infection control team should be involved in providing specific advice appropriate to the nature of the infection identified. This may involve contact tracing people who have been in contact with her, for example, if meningococcus is isolated, for prophylactic treatment (RCOG 2012b).

REFLECTION ON THE TRIGGER SCENARIO

Look back on the trigger scenario at the start of the chapter.

> *Julie phoned labour ward triage complaining of abdominal pain and just not feeling well. She was 28 weeks pregnant, expecting her second baby. Kim, the midwife, ran through the routine questions, 'Have you had any bleeding, any loss of fluid...?' Julie said that she thought she had leaked some urine 3 days ago and had felt damp ever since, but thought that was because the baby was pressing on her bladder. Kim said, 'I want you to make your way into the unit so we can check you and your baby over'.*

The scenario is one that any midwife working in a triage capacity might encounter. Midwives need to know what elements of a clinical history might give cause for concern. Now that you are familiar with the signs and symptoms of sepsis you should have insight into how the scenario relates to the evidence. The jigsaw model will now be used to explore the trigger scenario in more depth.

Effective communication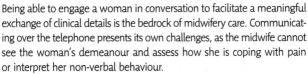

Being able to engage a woman in conversation to facilitate a meaningful exchange of clinical details is the bedrock of midwifery care. Communicating over the telephone presents its own challenges, as the midwife cannot see the woman's demeanour and assess how she is coping with pain or interpret her non-verbal behaviour.

Questions that arise from the scenario might include: How had Julie found the correct telephone number to ring? When had this been communicated to her and by whom? Had any circumstances caused Julie to delay making contact with the maternity unit? If so, what might those have been and how could they be avoided in the future?

Woman-centred care

When a woman makes contact with her maternity care provider she must be sure that the focus is on her needs and those of her baby. The midwife needs to listen attentively to her concerns and be able to adapt her care to meet them. No two women are the same, and what one woman anticipates with joy may make another tremble with fear. Questions that arise from the scenario might include: What can Kim do to ensure that Julie feels treated with kindness and compassion? Are there any elements of the documentation of care that might facilitate Julie engaging in her care as an equal partner? Did Kim consider how asking Julie to attend the hospital might affect her role as mother to her other child? Who would bring her in to hospital? Does she have her own transport? Who might accompany her and provide her with emotional support?

Using best evidence

Knowledge is increasing continuously about the recognition and management of sepsis. It is therefore vital that clinical guidelines reflect the most recent evidence base. There are a range of sources of evidence that are of particular value to the management of serious maternal illness, especially the annual confidential enquiries into maternal death. Questions that arise from the scenario might include: What protocol is being used to assess if Julie is at risk of sepsis? Is this one that is used throughout the trust or is it specific to maternity care? How has learning for the most recent confidential enquiry into maternal death been cascaded to the maternity care team? Who is responsible for ensuring that guidelines and protocols reflect best practice where you work?

Professional and legal issues

Midwives have a duty of care to the women they look after and this must be reflected in their approach to all women who present to maternity services. Midwives must take a comprehensive history from the woman or her relatives if she is unwell, and ensure that they escalate concerns to the appropriate medical team. Questions that arise from the scenario might include: What action should Kim take if Julie refuses to come to the maternity unit for care? What action should Kim take if Julies agrees to attend, but then does not arrive? In what circumstances can health professionals provide care without the woman's consent? Can Julie refuse treatment for a life-threatening illness?

Team working

To complement the advancement of new knowledge, it is essential that the maternity care team have opportunities to learn and practise together to ensure they are all up to speed with the latest techniques. It is also important that they recognize each other's roles in the management of a seriously ill woman and can complement each other's capabilities to maximize the potential for a positive outcome. Questions that arise from the scenario might include: How many professionals might potentially be involved in Julie's care if she is suspected of septicaemia on admission? Who would be responsible for initiating cardiopulmonary resuscitation (CPR) if Julie suddenly collapsed? What opportunities do the team members have to practise emergency drills together?

Clinical dexterity

When Julie arrives on the labour ward it is essential that she is cared for by a team who have the necessary skills to make an accurate assessment of her physiological status. Not only must the healthcare practitioners be able to undertake the necessary observations, but they also need to know when they fall outside of normal parameters and what they might be reflecting. Questions that arise from the scenario might include: Who will be taking Julie's observations when she arrives at the maternity unit? Who is responsible for acting on the results? What blood tests might be requested by the medical team and who will take them? By what means will the well-being of Julie's baby be determined? How will her neurological status be assessed and by whom?

Models of care

There are a range of models of care that women can access depending on their current health and well-being and current and previous medical and obstetric history. Many women are eligible for midwifery-led care at the point of booking; however, this may change as their pregnancy progresses. Women who have known risk factors may be booked for consultant-led or maternity team care at the outset. Questions that arise from the scenario might include: Has Julie's pregnancy been complication-free until this point? Is she booked for midwifery-led care and if so is this in a stand-alone or along-side facility? Where will she attend for her assessment when she feels unwell? Will she meet a midwife she has previously met? How will her pathway be changed if she requires consultant care in the future?

Safe environment

When sepsis is suspected it is essential that the woman is cared for in a place where she can receive life-saving treatment and care, and therefore she should be directed to an acute emergency setting. There should be no delay in commencing antibiotic therapy when sepsis may be the cause of a woman's ill health. Questions that arise from the scenario might include: How are staff caring for the woman protected from the risk of infection? What facilities are there where you work to care for a woman who might need to be nursed in isolation? How is contaminated waste disposed of? How can staff protect both themselves and the women they care for from the spread of infectious diseases, especially in the winter months?

Promotes health

Sepsis is a life-threatening condition but one that can potentially be avoided if women and their families are informed of the signs and symptoms to look out for. Women who have had a baby are more at risk because of the potential for pathogens to enter the blood stream through the placental site or traumatized genital tract, but they can take preventative measures to reduce their individual risk. Questions that arise from the scenario might include: Had Julie been aware that a 'loss of fluid' might be a sign that her waters had broken? How could this information be best made available to women? What platforms do the maternity services where you work use to promote health and well-being to their patients? What public health campaigns can you remember in relation to health in pregnancy and why?

Further scenarios

The following scenarios enable you to consider how specific situations influence the care the midwife provides. Use the jigsaw model to explore the issues raised in the scenario.

Cassie, a third-year student midwife, approached her mentor Sue and said, 'Is it OK if I pop down to the flu clinic later and have my flu vaccine?' Sue said, 'I don't know why you are bothering with that; my sister had the vaccine last year and she still got flu'.

Practice point

Influenza is a serious infection for anyone and can lead to serious complications and even death, particularly in those who are most vulnerable. Flu vaccination is offered to all pregnant women, at any gestation, each flu season. However, there is evidence that some frontline healthcare workers are reluctant to take up their opportunity to be protected from the virus and thus prevent spread of infection to their patients and their own families and colleagues; in 2017 to 2018 the uptake was 63.9% (Public Health England 2018).

Questions that arise from the scenario might include:

+ What are the contraindications to receiving the seasonal flu vaccine?
+ Is it a live vaccine?
+ Can the flu vaccine make you ill?
+ How long does it take to become effective?
+ What strains of influenza are covered in the vaccine?
+ Why are pregnant women more vulnerable to seasonal influenza and its consequences?
+ How is it administered to pregnant women?

Sabida was unwell with diarrhea and vomiting 5 days after having a normal birth. Lucy, the midwife, was reassured that her observations were normal. Over the next few days Sabida's condition deteriorated and she collapsed at home. Her mother called 999 for an ambulance and Sabida was admitted to the Accident and Emergency Department, where septic shock was diagnosed.

Practice point

When a woman is unwell, either when pregnant or postnatally, her condition must be closely monitored, as she is particularly vulnerable to infection and the development of sepsis. A comprehensive set of observations including temperature, pulse, respiration rate, blood pressure and mental state should inform the assessment. It is important to note that a MEOWS score alone should not be the only means of coming to a judgement about a woman's health or the only means for escalating concern (Knight et al 2017). Sepsis can also present with hypothermia, and it is important that local guidelines support a detailed postnatal assessment, followed by clear lines of escalation when a woman is unwell.

Questions that arise from the scenario might include:

+ What other considerations could Lucy have taken into account when assessing Sabida's health status on day 5?
+ What is the likely cause of her severe infection?
+ Who should now be involved in her care?
+ What investigations will be made?
+ What treatment will Sabida receive?
+ What information should be sought from her mother?
+ What are Sabida's chances of survival from septic shock?

Conclusion

Sepsis is a life-threatening condition triggered by the body's response to infection. With swift and appropriate investigation and treatment, women have a good chance of surviving to care for their baby and the midwife can play a key role in recognizing the condition and escalating her concerns. All maternity services should have a robust sepsis guideline in place complemented with screening tools and documentation that assist in this process.

Resources

All-Wales consensus policy exemplar guide: Sepsis in Pregnancy. Available at: http://www.1000livesplus.wales.nhs.uk/sitesplus/documents/1011/FINAL%20 Sepsis%20PEG%20NOV%202012.pdf.

NHS England, 2014. Patient Safety Alert: Resources to support the prompt recognition of sepsis and the rapid initiation of treatment. Available at: http:// www.england.nhs.uk/wp-content/uploads/2014/09/psa-sepsis.pdf.

Scone, G., Berghella, V., 2016. Antenatal corticosteroids for lung maturity. Available at: http://www.bmj.com/content/bmj/355/bmj.i5044.full.pdf.

Rhodes, A., et al., 2017. Surviving sepsis campaign. Available at: http://www .survivingsepsis.org/Guidelines/Pages/default.aspx.

The UK sepsis trust: Screening and action tool. Available at: https://sepsistrust.org/ wp-content/uploads/2017/08/ED-adult-NICE-Final-1107.pdf.

The UK sepsis trust: Inpatient maternal sepsis tool. Available at: https:// sepsistrust.org/wp-content/uploads/2017/08/Inpatient-maternal-NICE-Final-1107-2.pdf.

References

Knight, M., Kenyon, S., Brocklehurst, P., et al.; on behalf of MBRRACE – UK, eds, 2014. Saving lives, improving mothers' care: lessons learned to inform future maternity care from the UK and Ireland Confidential Enquiries into Maternal Deaths and Morbidity 2009–12. Oxford: National Perinatal Epidemiology Unit, University of Oxford.

Knight, M., Nair, M., Tuffnell, D., et al., (Eds.) on behalf of MBRRACE-UK. Saving Lives, Improving Mothers' Care - Surveillance of maternal deaths in the UK 2012-14 and lessons learned to inform maternity care from the UK and Ireland Con dential Enquiries into Maternal Deaths and Morbidity 2009-14. Oxford: National Perinatal Epidemiology Unit, University of Oxford 2016. https://www.npeu.ox.ac.uk/downloads/files/mbrrace-uk/reports/MBRRACE-UK%20 Maternal%20Report%202016%20-%20website.pdf.

Knight, M., Nair, M., Tuffnell, D., et al.; on behalf of MBRRACE – UK, 2017. Saving lives, improving mothers' care: lessons learned to inform maternity care from the UK and Ireland Confidential Enquiries into Maternal Deaths and Morbidity 2013–15. Oxford: National Perinatal Epidemiology Unit, University of Oxford.

Knowles, S., O'Sullivan, N., Meenan, A., et al., 2015. Maternal sepsis incidence, aetiology and outcome for mother and fetus: a prospective study. BJOG 122, 663–671.

NHS England, 2014. Patient Safety Alert: Resources to support the prompt recognition of sepsis and the rapid initiation of treatment. Available at: http://www.england.nhs.uk/wp-content/uploads/2014/09/psa-sepsis.pdf.

National Institute for Health and Care Excellence (NICE), 2016, updated 2017. Sepsis: recognition, diagnosis and early management. NICE clinical guideline 51. Available at: https://www.nice.org.uk/guidance/ng51.

Public Health England, 2018. Seasonal influenza vaccine uptake amongst frontline healthcare workers (HCWs) in England. Available at: https://www.gov.uk/government/uploads/system/uploads/attachment_data/file/676412/HCWs_Seasonal_Flu_Vaccine_December_Report_2017.pdf.

Rhodes, A., Evans, L.E., Alhazzani, W., et al., 2017. Surviving sepsis campaign: international guidelines for management of sepsis and septic shock: 2016. Intensive Care Med. 43, 304–377.

Roberts, N., Hooper, G., Lorencatto, F., et al., 2017. Barriers and facilitators towards implementing the Sepsis Six care bundle (BLISS-1): a mixed methods investigation using the theoretical domains framework. Scand. J. Trauma Resusc. Emerg. Med. 25, doi:10.1186/s13049-017-0437-2.

Royal College of Obstetricians and Gynaecologists (RCOG), 2010. Green-top Guideline No. 7: Antenatal corticosteroids to reduce neonatal morbidity and mortality. Available at: https://www.glowm.com/pdf/Antenatal%20Corticosteroids%20to%20Reduce%20Neonatal%20Morbidity.pdf.

Royal College of Obstetricians and Gynaecologists (RCOG), 2012a. Green-top Guideline No. 64a: Bacterial sepsis in pregnancy. London: Royal College of Obstetricians and Gynaecologists.

Royal College of Obstetricians and Gynaecologists (RCOG), 2012b. Green-top Guideline No. 64b: Bacterial sepsis following pregnancy. London: Royal College of Obstetricians and Gynaecologists.

Saccone, G., Berghella, V., 2016. Antenatal corticosteroids for maturity of term or near term fetuses: systematic review and meta-analysis of randomized controlled trials. BMJ 355, i5044. doi:10.1136/bmj.i5044. bmj.i5044.full.pdf.

Say, L., Chou, D., Gemmill, A., et al., 2014. Global causes of maternal death: a WHO systematic analysis. Lancet Glob. Health 2, e323–e333.

UK Sepsis Trust, 2016. Maternal sepsis toolkits. Available at: http://sepsistrust.org/clinical-toolkit/.

UK Sepsis Trust, 2018. Home page https://sepsistrust.org.

Vaught, A., 2018. Maternal sepsis. Semin. Perinatol. 42, 9–12.

Waechter, J., Kumar, A., Lapinsky, S.E., et al., 2014. Interaction between fluids and vasoactive agents on mortality in septic shock: a m UK Sepsis Trust ulticenter, observational study. Crit. Care Med. 42, 2158–2168.

World Health Organisation (WHO), 2017. Statement on maternal sepsis. Geneva: World Health Organisation.

Page numbers followed by "*f*" indicate figures, "*t*" indicate tables, and "*b*" indicate boxes.